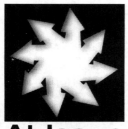

At Issue

Superfoods

Other Books in the At Issue Series:

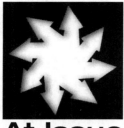

At Issue

▌Superfoods

Roman Espejo, Book Editor

GREENHAVEN PRESS
A part of Gale, Cengage Learning

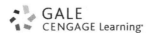

GALE
CENGAGE Learning·

Farmington Hills, Mich • San Francisco • New York • Waterville, Maine
Meriden, Conn • Mason, Ohio • Chicago

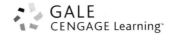

Judy Galens, *Manager, Frontlist Acquisitions*

For more information, contact:
Greenhaven Press
27500 Drake Rd.
Farmington Hills, MI 48331-3535
Or you can visit our Internet site at gale.cengage.com

For product information and technology assistance, contact us at

Gale Customer Support, 1-800-877-4253
For permission to use material from this text or product, submit all requests online at www.cengage.com/permissions

Further permissions questions can be e-mailed to permissionrequest@cengage.com

Articles in Greenhaven Press anthologies are often edited for length to meet page requirements. In addition, original titles of these works are changed to clearly present the main thesis and to explicitly indicate the author's opinion. Every effort is made to ensure that Greenhaven Press accurately reflects the original intent of the authors. Every effort has been made to trace the owners of copyrighted material.

LIBRARY OF CONGRESS CATALOGING-IN-PUBLICATION DATA

Superfoods / Roman Espejo, book editor.
    pages cm. -- (At issue)
Includes bibliographical references and index.
ISBN 978-0-7377-7412-2 (hardcover) -- ISBN 978-0-7377-7413-9 (pbk.)
1. Nutrition. 2. Health--Nutritional aspects. I. Espejo, Roman, 1977- editor.
RA784.S858 2016
 613.2--dc23
                        2015025548

Printed in Mexico
1 2 3 4 5 6 7 19 18 17 16

Contents

Introduction

It's hard to keep up with what's being hailed as the next big superfood. Take, for instance, a sampling of headlines found at the beginning of 2015: "9 New Superfoods You'll Be Eating in 2015," "New Celebrity Superfood Faves of 2015," "The Hot New Superfoods and Fads for 2015," "Over Kale? Here Are the New Superfoods of 2015," and "Forecast: Seeds, Nuts Top 'Superfoods' for 2015." It's just as hard to keep up with those foods that may be already passé. "2014's favorites were chia seeds, quinoa, sweet potatoes, salmon, kale and goji berries among others," writes Racha Adib, a dietitian based in Beirut, Lebanon. "While you should keep these superfoods handy, let's take a look at what 2015 has in store for us."[1]

Amaranth is one of the foods that Adib shortlists as the next superfood superstar. It's an ancient grain that was domesticated up to eight thousand years ago by the Aztecs. "Why [is it] trending? It's packed with protein of unusually high quality and it's gluten-free—a great option for people with celiac disease and gluten intolerances,"[2] she says. In fact, its protein content hovers around 13 percent, much higher than other grains. "You may hear the protein in amaranth referred to as 'complete' because it contains lysine, an amino acid missing or negligible in many grains,"[3] states the Whole Grains Council. Another touted benefit is that it's healthful for the heart. "Amaranth has shown potential as a cholesterol-lowing whole grain in several studies," adds the council.

1. Racha Adib, "New Superfoods on the Chopping Block: What Will Trend in 2015?," *Al Arabiya News*, January 8, 2015. http://english.alarabiya.net/en/life-style/healthy-living /2015/01/08/New-superfoods-on-the-chopping-block-What-will-trend-in-2015-.html.
2. Ibid.
3. Whole Grains Council, "Amaranth—May Grain of the Month," wholegrainscouncil .org (accessed May 16, 2015). http://wholegrainscouncil.org/whole-grains-101 /amaranth-may-grain-of-the-month-0.

Coconut palm sugar is another superfood that Adib says may start trending. Derived from the sap of flower buds of coconut palms, it has been used as a sweetener in Indonesia and the Philippines for millennia. "According to the Philippine Coconut Authority, coconut sugar has a lower Glycemic Index (35) compared to table sugar (60), making it a healthier alternative especially for Diabetics, but more studies are needed before making any conclusions,"[4] she observes. Plus, coconut palm sugar is reported to be healthier than cane sugar. "[C]oconut sugar is 70 to 79 percent sucrose and only three percent to nine percent each of fructose and glucose. This is an advantage, because you want to keep your consumption of fructose as low as possible, and cane sugar is 50 percent fructose,"[5] maintains Andrew Weil, founder, professor, and director of the Arizona Center for Integrative Medicine at the University of Arizona.

As for greens, Adib forecasts that dandelion may trump kale as the leafy superfood du jour. "Like other greens, they're a great source of antioxidants and a wide array of vitamins—a great way to support your diet as opposed to vitamin supplements. They also contain a lot of iron and fiber,"[6] she says. Dandelion greens are eaten as a salad and added as a key ingredient to juice cleanses. "The herb stimulates the flow of bile from the liver into the gall bladder, making dandelion a key ingredient in liver cleanse formulas. It helps to break down liver fats and is an effective diuretic,"[7] states Donna Earnest Pravel for the website Natural News. Furthermore, it may even have powerful cancer-fighting properties. "The scientific community has been frenetically studying dandelion recently,

4. Op. cit.
5. Andrew Weil, "Is Coconut Sugar a Healthier Sweetener?," www.drweil.com, August 12, 2013. http://www.drweil.com/drw/u/QAA401323/Is-Coconut-Sugar-a-Healthier -Sweetener.html.
6. Op. cit.
7. Donna Earnest Pravel, "Dandelion Gets Scientific Acceptance as an Antioxidant and 'Novel' Cancer Therapy," Natural News, March 31, 2012. http://www.naturalnews.com /035418_dandelion_cancer_therapy_herbs.html#ixzz3aMK1LXFh.

due to encouraging evidence that dandelion suppresses the growth and invasive behavior in several types of cancer," Pravel continues.

And how about the next superfruit? Adib nominates baobab, a tangy, gourd-like fruit that grows from the baobab tree in Africa and is valued for its medicinal properties. "Baobab contains six times as much vitamin C as oranges, twice as much calcium as milk, and it's also high in magnesium, iron, fiber, and antioxidants," she says. "Moreover, it has prebiotic qualities that can stimulate the 'good bacteria' in your gut and helps you maintain a healthy digestive system."[8] Everywhere else in the world, it's available as a jam and in powder form. "Baobab powder is . . . considered to be a great rehydration agent due to the high electrolyte profile, namely potassium and magnesium,"[9] writes Amy Crawford, founder of the *Holistic Ingredient* blog in Australia. "In addition these electrolytes and iron are all important alkalising minerals to promote correct body pH."

Regardless of which obscure food becomes the next must-have for health-conscious shoppers, it's clear that superfoods are appearing at more supermarket aisles and restaurant menus across the nation—whether or not they have nutritional superpowers. Indeed, in 2014, the market for these so-called nutritional foods was projected to grow to $130 billion in 2015. This volume, *At Issue: Superfoods*, examines such questions as why superfoods are so popular, whether superfoods really are good for you, and whether some superfoods are harmful to the environment. In the process, the authors of the following viewpoints take a look—and a bite out of—the health and wellness claims surrounding these fruits, vegetables, roots, seeds, and grains.

8. Op. cit.
9. Amy Crawford, "Superfood Feature: The Health Benefits of Baobab (New to Aussie Shores!)," www.theholisticingredient.com, October 10, 2014. http://www.theholisticingredient.com/blogs/wholesome-living/13589970-superfood-feature-the-health-benefits-of-baobab-new-to-aussie-shores.

1

Superfoods Have Significant Health Benefits

Josh Axe

Based in Nashville, Tennessee, Josh Axe is a physician, nutritionist, and founder of the Exodus Health Center. He also hosts Transform Your Health, *a weekly podcast.*

Superfoods are fruits, vegetables, and other natural foods dense in nutrients with proven health benefits. Eaten in combination, they can help individuals achieve a variety of goals, such as boosting weight loss, detoxing the body, and improving athletic performance. For instance, a study demonstrated that participants who ate African mango lost twenty-eight pounds more than those in the placebo group. Containing the same five electrolytes in human blood at the same levels, coconut juice is regarded as "nature's sports drink;" it also supports the immune system and fights off bacterial, viral, and fungal infections. And kale is the "king of the vegetable kingdom," packed with nutrients such as calcium, lutein, and vitamin B6—not calories—that exceed daily requirements.

Isn't it frightening to learn a loved one has a serious health problem like cancer, heart disease or diabetes? Five of six Americans die of heart disease or cancer, diabetes has tripled in the past ten years and by 2025 it's estimated that 50% of all Americans will be obese! People are in great danger today and desperately need a hero. . . . That hero is superfood.

What bodily villain are you battling? Weight Gain? Lack of Energy? Digestive Problems? No matter the issue, Superfoods can help you win!

Superfoods can help you conquer and achieve your health goals. Maybe you've tried every weight loss program, product, and pill on the planet, but the weight won't come off or it just keeps coming back. I have some great news for you!

I'm Dr. Josh Axe, and I'm here to help you become a super-you! I've seen thousands of people achieve their health goals through my radio show, books, and seminars. Everyone from stay-at-home moms to Olympic level athletes. I'm also a wellness physician and triathlete, but mostly I'm passionate about helping people transform their health and lives.

Are you ready to become a super-you?

Mom's Victory with Superfoods

Seventeen years ago my mom was diagnosed with breast cancer. That was a crazy reality for my family at the time because she was a gym teacher, swim instructor and an active mom who looked healthy. How could someone so active end up with cancer at forty? I was thirteen years old and remember asking myself this question, but having no answer.

My mom made a trip to the doctor where they recommended surgery and chemotherapy. Taking their advice, she went through all the traditional medical treatments. I still remember watching her hair fall out and thinking she had aged twenty years in two weeks after going through her chemo treatments. She pressed on through her treatments, like so many do today, and after battling for months she was diagnosed as cancer free and "healthy".

Sadly, even though she was diagnosed as being healthy after her treatments, she was sicker than ever. My mom struggled with chronic fatigue, depression, constipation and was sick all the time. She continued to have these problems for another ten years until one day I received a call from her. She'd just been told by her doctor that they found a 2.5 cm mass on her lungs, and from the scan, they believed it was cancer. They were recommending surgery and radiation, but this time she wanted to do something more natural.

Superfoods are natural, nutrient-dense compounds that contain high concentrations of essential nutrients with proven health benefits.

Rather than going the traditional medical route, she decided to follow my advice and take a natural approach. The biggest thing my mom changed was her diet. Previously, she thought the three main food groups were fast, frozen and instant. We changed that to kefir, kale and blueberries!

She went back for a checkup four months later, and to the doctor's amazement, the tumors had shrunk in half. One year later the tumors were completely gone! She needed a super-hero and we give all the glory to God for healing her, but we know that God created Superfoods to give her health back. Today she's in the best shape of her life.

She actually just raced her first 5K last year and finished second in her age group at fifty-eight years old! She went from supersick to superstar by eating superfoods. Can you see where superfoods could possibly help a loved one you know? Wouldn't it be of great value to them for you to share this information? . . .

What Are Superfoods?

Superfoods are natural, nutrient-dense compounds that contain high concentrations of essential nutrients with proven health benefits. They're high in vitamins, minerals, omega-3 fatty acids, probiotics, or antioxidants . . . just to name a few!

Over the past several years I've worked with a range of Olympic level athletes, and they all have the same thing in common . . . they're simply the best at what they do! I like to think of superfoods like Olympic competitors. If you're picking someone to be on your relay for swimming, do you want Joe Schmoe, who's never swam a day in his life, or Michael Phelps? It's obvious, [Olympic swimmer] Michael Phelps is a superior athlete and if you want to win, you want him on your team. It's the same with food.

If you want to age slower and live longer, you can pick donuts or blueberries to be on your team. If you want to win, go with blueberries because they have super antioxidants for anti-aging. I'm not saying you can eat a specific superberry once a day, followed by a double bacon cheeseburger, and still expect peak results. Superfoods work better as a team. Like [superheroes] the Avengers, X-Men, or PowerRangers by their powers combined. You can achieve super health results by combining certain superfoods together.

African Mango + Amasai + Chia = Super Weight Loss

What's your biggest health goal? Is it to lose weight, detox, age slower, build muscle, or increase athletic performance? Depending on what type of super results you want to see you're going to need a super plan. I know everyone has different health goals so I created 4 tracks for you to follow.

By eating the right superfoods, you won't just lose weight, but you'll be changing your life, your legacy, and changing your world!

I divided the superfoods into four sections, but all these superfoods can help you in all areas. For instance, the superfood amasai helps you lose body fat, build muscle, age slower, AND detox! I personally consume all the superfoods, so read through each section, then pick your plan at the end, Ready? Up, up, and away!

1. Weight Loss

2. Detox

3. Anti-Aging

4. Muscle Building

The statistics are stunning! 34% of Americans are obese and 32% are overweight. That means exactly 2/3 of Americans need to lose weight. Obesity has doubled since 1980 (*National Center for Health Statistics*). 32% of kids are overweight and 16% of American children are already obese (*Center for Disease Control, 2009*)!

We don't just need to lose weight to look good in a swimsuit, we need to lose weight to live and fulfill our God-given missions. Research shows that obesity doubles your risk of heart failure and triples the risk of breast cancer in women! The average middle age weight gain of 22 pounds increases your risk of a heart attack by 75%. But think about the flip side,

> If you lose 22 pounds, you decrease your risk of heart attack by 75% and risk of cancer by 50% (*Okinawa Diet 2004, Bradley*)!

By eating the right superfoods, you won't just lose weight, but you'll be changing your life, your legacy, and changing your world!

So let's jump into the nutrients that have been scientifically proven to help your body burn fat and lose weight.

African Mango

African Mango can help you lose weight in a flash! The powerful benefits of African Mango are now well publicized thanks to [television host] Dr. Oz. Recently, he featured it on the *Oprah Winfrey Show*, and extolled the virtues of this superfood as a weight loss aid and natural fat burner.

In a controlled study published in the *Journal of Nutrition*, 2008, humans taking this new compound lost 28 pounds over a 10-week period, compared to less than 3 pounds in the placebo group. Different than other weight loss studies that mandate at least some moderation in food intake, these study participants did not alter their diet in any way.

The specific compound in African mango which supports weight loss is called irvingia. This compound has shown better weight loss results than any hormone, drug or food in medical history!

Even if you don't need to lose weight, African mango is highly beneficial as it contains nutrients that naturally help lower LDL [low-density lipoprotein] cholesterol.

Recent research is proving that certain types of saturated fat are actually good and can help your body burn fat and lose weight.

The African mango is found in Cameroon, Africa, where its fruit and seeds have been used for hundreds of years for their medical benefits. Other names for African mango are "irvingia gaconesis" while natives call it "dikka nuts".

African mango (irvingia) works in four fantastic ways:

1. Works with adiponectin to increase insulin sensitivity.

2. Balances the hormone Leptin which signals your brain to burn fat.

3. Decreases the amount of blood glucose that turns into fat.

4. Blocks the enzyme amylase from digesting starches that would have otherwise become sugar.

In the two most popular clinical studies done on irvingia (African mango) 150mg was taken twice daily and participants lost 12.8 pounds in four weeks and 28 pounds in ten weeks. I personally drink one serving daily with 150mg of African mango 30–45 minutes before meals, or two times daily to get the fantastic four results of African mango.

Coconut

Ever wonder how superheroes like Wonder Woman always look so good in spandex? It could be from consuming coconut. For years coconut has taken the blame for containing saturated fat. But recent research is proving that certain types of saturated fat are actually good and can help your body burn fat and lose weight!

Coconut contains healthy fats called medium chain fatty acids (MCTs). A study published in the *International Journal of Obesity* found that MCTs increase lipid (fat) oxidation, which means coconut will burn up excess calories and help you lose weight! Coconut has also been shown to reduce cholesterol, triglycerides, phospholipids and LDL cholesterol levels.

If coconut oil is taken at the same times as omega-3 fatty acids it can make them twice as effective, as they are readily available to be digested and used by the body.

According to a study at California State University, grass-fed beef and dairy contain three times more CLA than grain-fed beef and dairy.

Athletes have found that coconut liquid enhances their performance and hydration. NBA [National Basketball Association] superstar Kevin Garnett has partnered with [singer] Madonna to invest in a coconut water company, seeing it as "nature's sports drink"! Coconut liquid has the same five electrolytes in the same levels as human blood: sodium, phosphorous, calcium, magnesium and potassium, making it a great superfood contender.

The MCTs found in coconut are also used in popular muscle building products like Muscle Milk. Most companies use processed MCTs, but if you eat real coconut, you're getting high quality MCTs. They aren't just good for burning fat, they're also great for building muscle.

Coconut also improves digestion as it helps the body absorb fat-soluble vitamins, calcium and magnesium. It's a powerful aid to your immune system and can fight off bacteria, viruses and fungal overgrowth such as Candida. When buying coconut oil, make sure to get "unrefined". I think Coconut might be the secret for how [actor] Christian Bale got those abs for the Batman movies!

Green-Fed Dairy (CLA)

Want to know where [superhero] Mighty Mouse got all his Mojo? Well, what do mice love most? Cheese! Cheese and other dairy products like amasai, milk and butter contain CLA (conjugated linoleic acid), a fatty acid that burns fat. But, it can't be just any cheese or dairy product. In order for dairy to have high amounts of CLA, the cow must be fed grass and not grains.

Green-fed is the highest standard and typically contains the largest amount of CLA. According to a study at California State University, grass-fed beef and dairy contain three times more CLA than grain-fed beef and dairy.

It's been shown to promote weight loss, burn fat, fight cancer, and even reduce the risk of heart disease, according to the *American Journal of Clinical Nutrition*, May 2010.

A study out of the *Journal of Animal Sciences* found that grass-fed cows may produce 300–500% more CLA than cows fed corn and grains.

Over thirty-five clinical studies have been done on CLA displaying its amazing ability to aid the body in burning fat and building muscle! There are sixteen different types of CLA and most commercial supplements found in health food stores today contain only two! You could spend $50+ a month on this supplement, however, the best source for CLA is to consume high quality grass-fed or green-fed meat and dairy.

Cinnamon

Can you name a superfood that is very high in calcium (yet is not a dairy product), high in fiber, iron and manganese? The only food that ticks all these boxes is cinnamon. Even better, it is inexpensive, has no side effects, and has a host of health benefits. Its essential oils make it valued for its warming qualities as it aids fat burning as well.

A twelve-week study out of London found that Cinnamon drops A1c levels in diabetics by 7% (*Journal of British Diabetic Association*). The participants in the study took 2g of cinnamon daily and it not only helped with blood sugar, but it also significantly reduced blood pressure.

Another study found that cinnamon increased glucose metabolism by about twenty times, which would make a huge difference in your body being able to regulate blood sugar.

Though kale only has thirty-five calories per serving it is packed with calcium, magnesium, vitamin B6, lutein, and beta-carotene.

Cinnamon works in three different ways. First, it slows the emptying of your stomach to reduce sharp rises in blood sugar. Second, it increases insulin sensitivity. Third, cinnamon enhances your anti-oxidant defenses.

A recent study found that there are two antioxidants found in cinnamon called polyphenols and bioflavanoids, which may be responsible for all the health benefits. Antioxidants can work in many different ways like protecting your cells against free-radical damage that can cause aging. But these antioxidants seem to regulate blood sugar, which can help your body burn fat and lose weight! From all the research we've seen, cinnamon has been shown to help diabetics, lower blood pressure, and boost your metabolism! Who knew this sweet tasting herb could have such a sweet effect on your body!

Kale

It's a bird, it's a plane, no it's . . . Kale?! According to Joel Fuhrman, author of *Eat to Live*, kale is king in the vegetable kingdom. Though kale only has thirty-five calories per serving it is packed with calcium, magnesium, vitamin B6, lutein, and beta-carotene. Plus, it delivers 206% of the daily requirements of vitamin A, 134% of vitamin C, and 684% of vitamin K which helps build strong bones, improve vision, and aid in digestion!

Many people today spend time counting their calories when they should be counting their nutrients instead. Americans need more nutrient dense foods, and green leafy vegetables like kale are the most nutrient dense foods on the planet!

Results of a study in the *British Medical Journal* reviewed six studies covering more than 220,000 people, concluding that one and one half servings of green leafy vegetables per day lowered the risk of Type II diabetes by 14% and boosted metabolism.

Kale can be eaten raw or cooked and I recommend it sauteed in coconut oil with garlic, onions and sea salt, in a salad, or put into a green super smoothie. With numbers like these it's no wonder why kale is king in the vegetable kingdom. Start eating kale today to soar to new heights in health!

2

Superfoods That Don't Have Publicists

Ian Marber

Ian Marber studied nutrition at the Institute for Optimum Nutrition, founded "The Food Doctor," a nutritional consultancy, and writes on the subject of nutrition. He is a regular contributor to The Spectator.

The trend to label food items as superfoods is a marketing strategy used by companies to increase sales. Superfoods tend to be from exotic places and are artisanal, glamorous, or hard to find. However, there are readily available, less exotic superfoods that can be found locally, and usually less expensive.

Do you remember noni juice? No? Let me help you out. Noni, an exotic fruit, was proclaimed a superfood about 15 years ago, and was one of the first foods to receive that label. In 2011 there was coconut water, while in the last year or so chia seeds from Australia have taken over and are still doing well in health food shops.

But what makes a superfood, and who decides what qualifies? Although I'd like to think that there was a group of learned biochemists and nutrition geeks poring over the research before bestowing the title of 'superfood', the term is no more than smart marketing. In fact you could define a superfood as 'any food with a publicist'.

Ian Marber, "Superfoods That Don't Have Publicists," *The Spectator*, November 22, 2014.

While it's easy to be dismissive as a result, increasing awareness of what we eat is no bad thing. Marketing isn't always about getting us to buy pointless crap, it can be used for good too—consider the effects of the 'five a day' slogan. Even if we don't eat the recommended five servings of fruits and vegetables a day, most of us know that the guidance exists. Terming a food a superfood does encourage attention, from food writers and bloggers as well as buyers in supermarkets and, ultimately, consumers too.

PR doesn't come cheap, and superfoods tend to be pricey. The PR firm has an easier job when the food in question is from somewhere exotic, such as Tahiti in the case of noni juice. Ideally, it would have been favoured by local tribes for many thousands of years to give them energy to prepare them for battle or fight pain. If it has anything to do with fertility or sexual stamina, that's marketing gold.

Supermarkets stock significantly more individual items than any other type of shop and so a food needs to do something to get noticed.

When goji berries were first introduced into the UK, the PRs talked them up with references to Amazonian tribes (although I suspect the tribespeople would happily have traded their berries for some paracetamol). But clearly it worked, because goji were a big hit in 2007. These small orangey/red berries contain beta-carotene, vitamin C, zeaxanthin, lutein, essential fats, minerals—it's a long list—but while they are a good source of these nutrients, they are certainly not a unique source. They taste pleasant enough and if you have a poor diet, then adding a spoonful of these to a bowl of cereal would be helpful. But if you have a decent diet, they aren't life-changing. (Similarly, blueberries may be rich in phytochemicals, but adding them to a muffin or pancakes won't compensate for the refined flour and sugars.)

So provenance is a big factor in achieving superfood status. This means that broccoli, for example, does not have quite the same clout, though it is rich in a variety of nutrients including glucosinolates (also found in other cruciferous vegetables), from which isothiocyanates are made, which themselves can reduce inflammation as well as enhance liver detoxification. Broccoli also contains kaempferol, a flavanol that can help mediate allergic responses, as well as fibre, which offers a degree of protection against colon cancer and reduces LDL cholesterol.

Broccoli is reasonably priced too, unlike goji berries—but what it has in nutrients it lacks in not being artisanal, glamorous or hard to find (all of which are desirable properties in a superfood).

Food is unique in one aspect in that buying it is relentlessly repetitive. There is nothing else that we buy that we have to choose so frequently. Not clothing, fuel, books, movies, financial services, not even water—these are things we must purchase sometimes, but we make choices about what we want to eat several times a day. What's more, supermarkets stock significantly more individual items than any other type of shop and so a food needs to do something to get noticed.

What better way than to claim it has special properties? But there is an unexpected dark side to promoting foods in this way.

Take quinoa, a superfood from the Andes that enjoyed a huge increase in popularity during the 2000s, and has led to a larger percentage of crops from Bolivia and Peru being exported. Whereas the grain was once a staple food for locals, the popularity of quinoa in Europe and the US means that more is being sold abroad. At the same time imported food has become cheaper, and so refined flour imports are increasing to make up the shortfall. Not quite like for like then.

But don't be taken in by the marketing, as we have many less exotic and more readily available British products that, like broccoli, should be considered for superfood status. Whether it's rapeseed oil from Suffolk in place of olive oil, strawberries from Hampshire instead of goji, kale from Lincolnshire, apples from Somerset, salmon from Scotland or leeks from Wales—they all qualify. Even if we may not be able to pull that much glamour out of the hat when it comes to marketing, surely local is always super?

3

The Research on Superfoods Is Exaggerated by the Media

National Health Service

The National Health Service refers to the four public health-care systems in the United Kingdom.

Newspapers, magazines, and the Internet are full of headlines declaring the miraculous effects of so-called superfoods. Nonetheless, much of what the media reports is either inaccurate or counterproductive. The limitations of the research behind many articles about superfoods are rarely noted. For instance, a confounding factor—something other than the main factor being researched—may actually be responsible for the benefit instead of the superfood. Furthermore, other studies are plagued by subjects' inaccurate self-assessments or are based on animal or laboratory experiments that can't be replicated in humans. Therefore, readers must use common sense when encountering such research in the media and ask themselves if the association between a superfood and health outcome is plausible.

"Curry could save your life." "Beetroot can fight dementia." "Asthma risk linked to burgers." Every day there's a new crop of seemingly life-changing headlines about how the food we eat affects our health.

We all know that a good diet is an essential part of a healthy lifestyle, so it's not surprising that newspapers, magazines and the internet are full of stories about miracle superfoods and killer snacks.

Of course, there's more to it than that. There's a vast industry devoted to finding new ways to persuade us to eat this or that food and an army of scientists bent on exploring the links between what we eat and how healthy we feel.

Unfortunately, much of what is reported can be either inaccurate or unhelpful. The news is full of contradictory reports and often the same food is declared healthy one day and harmful the next.

Take alcohol. Sometimes it's reported to be good for your health, while other times it's bad. Some days we're told to drink in moderation, while on others even a single glass is too much.

Although some stories highlight the potential harms of particular foods, most proclaim benefits.

The facts about the latest dietary discoveries are rarely as simple as the headlines imply. Accurately testing how any one element of our diet may affect our health is fiendishly difficult. And this means scientists' conclusions, and media reports of them, should routinely be taken with a pinch of salt. . . .

Food stories are one of the most frequently occurring topics that Behind the Headlines covers, featuring in about a fifth of the 1,750 appraisals since mid-2007.

A quick analysis shows just how confusing these stories can be. Of the 1,750 Behind the Headlines appraisals carried out up to January 18, 2011, based on stories in the national press, 344 were about foods that had repercussions for health. We analysed those that reported on a single food or drink, grouping them into 106 single foodstuffs. Categorising these stories into whether the food was reported to be good for health or harmful gives a crude yet revealing indication of how food science is portrayed in the press. . . .

Although some stories highlight the potential harms of particular foods, most proclaim benefits.

When grouped as foodstuffs, 27 foods had been labelled harmful by headline writers, while 65 had been declared beneficial. Fourteen, however, have been labelled both healthy and harmful in different headlines. Chocolate, for example, can reportedly cause weak bones and depression, but other studies have claimed that it can also help fight cancer.

What Is a Superfood?

So more than half of the articles discussing a foodstuff focus on some sort of benefit.

But what really seems to capture the imagination of journalists and consumers is the idea that a single food, sometimes called a superfood, can confer remarkable health benefits.

There is no official definition of a superfood and the EU [European Union] has banned the use of the word on product packaging unless the claim is backed up by convincing research. A number of well-known brands have been forced to drop the description. However, there are still some proponents of the term, in spite of its loose definition.

News headlines, meanwhile, abound with claims that certain foods have super health benefits. Celery, broccoli, jam, popcorn and cereals have all been hyped as superfoods in the past couple of years. Other foods are said to be packed with chemicals that can ward off major killers such as cancer and heart disease.

Wine, for example, can allegedly:

- "add five years to your life"
- "help keep teeth healthy"
- "protect your eyes"
- make women "less likely to gain weight"

While broccoli can allegedly "undo diabetes damage", "stop breast cancer spreading" and "protect the lungs".

Even our beloved cuppa has been given superfood status. Black tea has been alleged to protect against heart disease. Green tea can supposedly cut the risk of prostate cancer. And it has been claimed that camomile can keep diabetes under control.

It's not uncommon for headlines to claim the most miraculous health benefit of all—that a food can save your life.

Miracle claims are also made for chocolate, including that a daily bar "can cut the risk of heart attack and stroke".

And it's not uncommon for headlines to claim the most miraculous health benefit of all—that a food can save your life. The following are all genuine claims from UK [United Kingdom] media from the past two years:

- "2½ bottles of wine a week can save your life"

- "A daily dose of garlic can save your life"

- "Just one bite of chocolate a day can help save your life"

- "Beetroot juice could save your life"

- "Curry could save your life"

You could be forgiven for thinking the secret of eternal life is a daily vindaloo, washed down with a glass of wine or two and a chocolate dessert.

The Trouble with Food Research

Of course, the truth is that these claims are almost always overstated. Unfortunately, research into the effects of single foods on our health is notoriously tricky to carry out. We have complex diets and it is difficult to disentangle the effects of one particular food or compound from all of the others we consume. This means that many of the studies behind the superfood claims have limitations. These limitations are rarely reported in the media, and even more rarely given their true significance.

Some of these limitations are discussed below. Knowing about them will help you to sort science fact from news fiction.

Many studies looking at foods rely on people being able to recall what they have been eating and drinking in some detail, sometimes several months or more in the past.

Confounding Factors

Confounding is a common problem in health research. Confounding is where something other than the main factor that is being assessed (a confounding factor) may be responsible for effects.

Take the story about half a glass of wine a day adding five years to your life. The results of this study of 1,373 Dutch men who were followed for over 40 years certainly sounded promising. The study found that men who consumed an average of about half a small glass of either red or white wine a day lived about five years longer than those who didn't drink alcohol. It also found a lower risk of death from cardiovascular disease among those who drank a small amount of wine compared with teetotallers. In humans, this type of study, called a cohort study, is often used to find out more about diet and health. Cohort studies enable researchers to follow large groups of people for many years to find out if a specific food or supplement is associated with a particular health outcome. A long follow-up period is particularly important when researchers are looking at the relationship between diet and outcomes such as cancer and heart disease.

The difficulty is that there are many things that can affect how long we might live or whether we're at risk of cardiovascular disease. They probably include, for example, social status, physical activity, body mass index (BMI) and the overall quality of our diet. Therefore, if the groups being compared (in this study those who drank a small amount of wine and teetotallers) differ in any of these other factors this could be contributing to the differences in lifespan, rather than just wine consumption.

Researchers call things that can affect the results of a study in this way confounders, and the best cohort studies adjust their findings to take into account as many confounders as possible. The wine study, for example, adjusted its findings for several possible confounders, such as smoking status, BMI, medical history and socioeconomic status. Surprisingly, however, it didn't adjust for how much physical activity the men did. If more wine drinkers than teetotallers exercised regularly, then this could be why the former lived longer than the latter.

A study that suggested that green tea could reduce the likelihood of developing prostate cancer had a similar weakness. It found that men who drank five cups of green tea a day were about half as likely to develop advanced prostate cancer as those who drank only one cup. This study involved nearly 66,000 men in Japan, who were followed for 14 years. It was a study with a large number of participants and a long follow-up, both of which are strengths. But it's possible that men who drink lots of green tea are also more likely to adhere to a traditional Japanese diet. This means diet may be a confounding factor. In fact, this is partly what the researchers found—that men who drank more green tea also ate more miso and soy, as well as fruit and vegetables. They also differed in other ways from men who drank less green tea. So it's difficult to say for certain whether the green tea is responsible for the lower risk of cancer or whether other elements in the diet were involved.

Inaccurate Memories

Many studies looking at foods rely on people being able to re-call what they have been eating and drinking in some detail, sometimes several months or more in the past. Recall bias is an important problem. Do you remember how many eggs you ate last year? Do you think your memory of those eggs would be affected if you found out you had high cholesterol? In the Dutch study of alcohol and mortality mentioned above, men were asked to recall how much they were eating and drinking up to a year ago. This is not unusual in studies of food. Esti-mating how much alcohol a person has consumed is especially tricky as the alcohol content varies between drinks. There are many reasons why people may look back with rose-tinted spectacles (and rosy cheeks) at their alcohol consumption and may underestimate the amount they consumed. Some may do this deliberately because they don't want to look bad when they complete their questionnaire.

Often, studies measure outcomes that aren't directly relevant to people's health.

Recall bias wouldn't be such a problem if it affected all people in a study equally, but often those with a particular outcome will remember their consumption differently from those who don't have that outcome. The eggs/high cholesterol example above is one, but the same may happen to people with food poisoning. People who have had food poisoning are much more likely to remember the evening out and the funny tasting curry than someone who didn't get ill. This inconsis-tency in recall depending on the outcome leads to bias in studies.

Additionally, what we eat and drink can vary from day to day and from year to year. So, if we are asked about our cur-rent eating habits, our answers may not be representative of what we have eaten throughout the rest of our lives. Food questionnaires often also ask about how many portions or cups of certain foods are eaten per week, and people may have different ideas about portion or cup sizes.

Proxy Outcomes

Often, studies measure outcomes that aren't directly relevant to people's health. Instead, they choose a proxy, which is something that is easier to test and which may be an indicator of a health benefit. The trouble is that media reports often confuse these proxy measures with the real thing.

Let's look at an example. A claim that omega-3 fats may be an "elixir of youth" was based on research in heart patients that didn't look primarily at patients' health, but at the length of telomeres, which are regions of DNA at the ends of chromosomes.

Telomeres shorten each time a cell divides, so telomere length is often used as a proxy measure for (an indicator of) biological ageing.

The study found that people with higher omega-3 levels in their blood also had less shortening of their telomeres. That's interesting, but it tells us nothing about whether omega-3 fats had any impact on the patients' health or on the cardiovascular disease process.

Similarly, one study that reportedly showed that oily fish could reduce memory loss did not measure people's memory. It scanned people's brains for areas starved of oxygen (called infarcts) and other abnormalities, to find out if there was any association between fish consumption and brain changes.

Eating fish three times a week was associated with a non-statistically significant reduction in risk of these brain abnormalities. Even if the difference had been significant, the study could not say whether oily fish prevents memory loss, as memory was not measured. Only a trial that directly measures people's memory can tell us about the link between oily fish and memory.

Animal and Laboratory Studies

Using a study in humans to link an indirect outcome measure to a disease is one thing, but many of the health stories reported in the press have not been carried out in people at all. Animal and laboratory studies are often used to test what researchers suspect to be the active components of foods, which might in time be developed into drug treatments or supplements.

Studies on cells or tissues in the laboratory may give useful clues to a food's properties, but they are often overinterpreted by the media.

There's been a lot of excitement, for example, about resveratrol, a compound found in red wine that has been shown to extend the life of yeasts, roundworms, fruit flies and also obese mice fed a high-calorie diet. Studies of this compound have suggested that resveratrol may cause cellular changes that have a positive effect on age-related processes, and may possibly have other benefits.

However, the doses of resveratrol used in lab studies may bear no relation to how much resveratrol humans can realistically get from drinking red wine. In one study, which found resveratrol helped stop abnormal growth of blood vessels in the eyes of mice, the human equivalent of the dose given would be several bottles of wine a day.

Before you reach for the resveratrol supplements (which do exist), bear in mind that just because this compound was associated with cellular changes in mice and some invertebrates, that doesn't mean it will have the same effect in humans. Animal studies are a valuable first step in finding out more about the active ingredients in a food or drink, but we need to wait for the results of clinical trials to find out if the same results hold true for humans.

Studies on cells or tissues in the laboratory may give useful clues to a food's properties, but they are often overinterpreted by the media. There is often a long way to go before we know whether lab findings could be relevant to humans eating food in real-life situations.

In one lab study that inspired the headline "Broccoli may undo diabetes damage", researchers applied sulforaphane, a compound found in broccoli, to human blood vessels incubated with sugar. Their aim was to find out whether sulforaphane could prevent damage to small blood vessels caused by high blood sugar (which can happen if you have diabetes). They found that sulforaphane did seem to protect cells from potentially damaging chemicals. This is an interesting finding, but a far cry from the claims of the news headline.

In another study, sulforaphane was applied to human breast cancer and mouse cancer cells in the laboratory and injected into mice with mammary gland tumours. The results suggested that the compound may be able to target cancer stem cells and stop them from dividing as much. This finding is promising and certainly warrants further research, but it would be misleading, possibly dangerous, to assume it means that eating broccoli can stop cancer in its tracks.

Who Gets It Wrong?

Sometimes it's not newspapers that are at fault in misinterpreting these kinds of studies, but researchers and press officers anxious to garner publicity. One study found that broccoli improved heart muscle function in rats whose hearts had been removed and subjected to a simulated heart attack. The title of the study called broccoli a "unique vegetable", when it is unknown if other vegetables might have the same result. It also implied that the results could apply to mammals generally, when that remains to be seen.

Sometimes, a suggested association between a food and a health outcome looks doubtful on the basis of common sense.

In such cases we have to ask ourselves whether the association seems plausible. For instance, in the study linking chocolate consumption to better cardiovascular health, people who ate the most chocolate had a 39% lowered risk of heart attack or stroke compared with those who ate the least chocolate. However, the difference in consumption between those who ate the most and those who ate the least chocolate was minimal: less than one small square (5g) of a 100g bar. Common sense tells us that this difference is unlikely to account for a 39% reduction in cardiovascular risk. The idea that helping yourself to a bar of chocolate a day will stop you having a heart attack or stroke may sound attractive, but this research does not provide any basis for it.

4

The Superfood Revolution

Nigel Huddleston

Nigel Huddleston is a journalist based in the United Kingdom.

From beetroot to lemongrass, mainstream food manufacturers are adding superfoods to their products to boost sales. Some include the term in the names, but most add superfoods to the recipes, relying on consumers to view the products as healthy without marketing them as health foods. Furthermore, the addition of superfoods to products enables brands to tap into the trend of natural ingredients. The impact on sales has been mixed; some brands have seen sales rise, while others have experienced falling sales. But as consumer interest in superfoods and health foods grows, manufacturers are already seeking out the next new super ingredient.

Beetroot and buffalo berries; chard and chia seeds; guarana and lemongrass. No, this isn't Gwyneth Paltrow's shopping list—these are just some of the new 'superfoods' mainstream FMCG players are putting into products to boost their functional credentials.

In March, Innocent launched a range of functional smoothies containing ingredients such as guarana, flax and echinacea; Tropicana has trialled an 'energising' juice with guarana since last year; and smaller brands are embracing functional superfoods by offering everything from beetroot sports bars to 'detoxifying' soups.

But how do such products sit with the strict health claims rules of the European Food Safety Authority (EFSA), which transformed the functional foods market when they came in force in 2012? And can superfoods really superpower functional sales?

Suppliers making claims about the functional properties of their products—whether linked to antioxidants, probiotics or more obscure areas such as the positive effect of almonds on erectile dysfunction—were forced to go back to the drawing board when EFSA started clamping down on health claims.

A number of suppliers and retailers have launched products with the term "superfoods" in their name.

Under the new rules, only a relatively narrow list of 222 approved claims is allowed (more recently expanded to 228). Crucially, that list does not currently include probiotics, meaning some of the biggest names in functional foods—such as Yakult and Danone's Actimel—have had to seriously overhaul their positioning in recent years. Actimel focuses more on vitamins and general wellbeing these days, while Yakult has steered away from specific gut health claims and adopted the more generic assertion that it contains "lots and lots of very good stuff".

EFSA's strict rules on health claims—and the bruising experience some major brands have had with them—are one of the reasons superfoods have become such an attractive option for the functional foods sector. The term 'superfoods' isn't regulated by EFSA; it's a marketing term, so suppliers have much more flexibility in how they use it to market their products and can respond more quickly to emerging functional food trends.

A number of suppliers and retailers have launched products with the term 'superfoods' in their name. For example,

Tesco offers a 'Super Food Salad' containing beans, lentils, spinach, beetroot and broccoli under its new My Fit Lifestyle range.

More commonly, however, superfoods are incorporated into recipes without the term itself appearing on packs. Instead, suppliers rely on consumers perceiving certain ingredients—such as berries, kale or beetroot—as especially healthy, creating a halo effect for the entire product without marketing having to be explicitly health-oriented.

Dairy brand The Collective is taking this approach. Its new yoghurt drinks contain ingredients that have a reputation as super-foods—such as oats and chia seeds—but it has steered clear of using the term itself. "There are strict regulations on naming products, so we've decided not to use the terms 'superfoods' or 'rich in antioxidants'," says head of NPD Fiona Cramp.

Others have gone for slight variations on the superfoods theme. First Milk's Team Sky range of high-protein smoothies and porridge includes a 'super fruit' flavour, and meat supplier Speyside has looked to bring the super-foods trend into burgers with the launch last year of Powerfoods—a range of lean beefburgers containing berries, oats and seeds.

While the 'superfood' concept is giving suppliers a bit more freedom in marketing terms, the limitations arising from the EFSA clampdown remain a major frustration for the category. "There are restrictions on health claims, which mean if a consumer has a particular ailment of need, a brand must rely on them to come to their own conclusions from the often limited on-pack information given," says Joanne Hayden, sales and marketing manager at Linwoods Health Foods.

Natural credentials

Adding superfoods to products also allows brands to tap growing consumer interest in natural ingredients.

Kantar research shows natural/unprocessed credentials are one of the key purchase drivers for consumers buying food and drink for health reasons, second only to general health benefits.

This trend is influencing NPD across the functional sector. In dairy, Volac is marketing its Upbeat drink partly on the fact it contains naturally derived protein and calcium.

Innocent and Tropicana are not the only major drinks players pinning their hopes on functional ingredients to boost sales.

Elsewhere, guarana is enjoying growing popularity, thanks to the naturally high levels of caffeine it contains. Late last year, PepsiCo began trialling Tropicana Energy—a blend of mango, guava, passion fruit and guarana, aimed at giving drinkers a "midmorning boost"—in Tesco. The product has since racked up just over £800,000 in sales.

Guarana also features in Innocent's new three-strong range of Super Smoothies, launched in March, which comes in Energise (containing strawberry, cherry and guarana); Defence (mango, pumpkin and echinacea); and Antioxidant (with kiwi, lime and wheatgrass).

The brand's hopes are high indeed. It is targetig sales of £30m within the first two years, with James Peach, UK smoothies manager at Innocent, adding: "We will see new trends coming from the US, particularly around premium fruit & veg juice."

Sales impact

Innocent and Tropicana are not the only major drinks players pinning their hopes on functional ingredients to boost sales. And not all are banking on superfoods—more conventional functional claims, such as around added vitamins, also remain big business.

Lucozade Revive, launched in March 2012, contains a blend of B vitamins and is marketed on its ability to assist the release of energy—a claim that is becoming more popular across the functional sector.

And Lucozade Sport's core marketing message was changed last year to focus on the product's ability to 'maintain hydration' and 'improve endurance performance'. The strategy seems to be working: IRI figures for the year to 29 March put sales of the brand up 9.5% on volumes up 8.6%.

By contrast, stablemate Ribena Plus has seen sales slide by 13.2% to £8.7m over the past year, despite being marketed on its vitamin content. Last month, Lucozade Ribena Suntory announced a TV campaign and redesign to boost sales. "The pack redesign showcases the 'no added sugar' message and additional nutrients," says category director Georgina Thomas.

Even with superfoods, super ingredients do not always translate into super sales. Last month Dairy Crest lost its last multiple listing for Clover Seedburst, after the spread—which contains 'seven healthy seeds and wholegrains'—hit just over £336,000 in sales in the year to 26 April. The dairy giant has had better success with more conventional functional claims around added vitamins and minerals: its Clover Additions range of functional spreads is now worth £2.6m and accounts for 3% of Clover sales.

But the continued success of some conventional functional claims is not to say the superfoods trend is about to run out of steam. Brands are already eyeing the next generation of super ingredients to add to their products.

Super seeds

Flax is one such ingredient. Innocent decided to add it to its Super Smoothies range, after research showed consumers were mixing regular smoothies with flax at home. Flax, along with other so-called 'super seeds' such as chia, are in high demand from health nuts because of their high content of dietary fibre and omega-3, as well as nutrients such as iron, zinc and calcium.

Linwoods claims its range of superfood meal supplements, which include milled organic flaxseed and chia seed, has seen value grow by 15%.

The time is right for suppliers and retailers to get behind seed-based products, believe experts.

And The Chia Company, which has seen sales leap in Australia and the US after TV ad campaigns, says it will be building on chia's popularity here in the UK with high-profile marketing this year.

The time is right for suppliers and retailers to get behind seed-based products, believe experts. "People are starting to become alert to the fact that omega-3 isn't just available through oily fish," says Debbie Dooly, marketing director at Chia Bia, which produces a range of seed mixes, biscuits and snack bars.

Other superfoods tipped for greatness include sprouted grains. These have been shown to have a positive impact on blood pressure, heart function and blood pressure, making them a key superfood to watch, according to Nick Barnard, co-founder of Rude Health. "We're planning a new range around sprouted grains in the autumn, which will be three ingredients and one new food product. It's the next big trend in functionality."

Tasneem Backhouse, sales & marketing director at EHL, is backing other, even more obscure foods. "Ancient grains have experienced a boom over the past five years," she says, pointing to teff and freekeh as ingredients that have surged in recent years, partly in response to growing demand for free-form foods.

With so many new superfoods to choose from, and con-sumer interest in healthy and functional eating on the rise, the brands will have plenty of opportunities to supercharge their products for many years to come.

5

More Restaurants Are Adding Superfoods to Their Menus

Bret Thorn

Based in New York City, Bret Thorn is senior editor of Nation's Restaurant News *and a food writer.*

More restaurants are sprinkling superfoods, which are high in nutrients and healthy compounds, onto their menus to stand out and generate sales. While once little-known ingredients like kale, quinoa, and açai are appearing at the biggest national chains, other operators are searching out those they predict will be part of the next wave of superfoods. Among these are tumeric (prized for its natural anti-inflammatory and antioxidant properties), chia seeds (noted for their high content of omega-3 oils and fiber), and exotic produce like mangosteen and maqui berries. However, restaurants can always rely on offering simple, fresh, and unprocessed fruits and vegetables, which are also superfoods.

As even the quick-service burger giants offer healthful menu items these days, it's harder for restaurants to stand out from the crowd with foods that will excite the growing numbers of health-conscious customers.

Many restaurants have started sprinkling their menus with more superfoods, that broad category of items with unusually high levels of antioxidants, protein, probiotics, omega-3 oils or other nutritious components.

Bret Thorn, "Superfoods to the Rescue: Concepts Use the Popular Category to Differentiate Healthful Fare, Generate Sales," *Nation's Restaurant News*, April 29, 2013. Copyright © 2013 Nation's Restaurant News. All rights reserved. Reproduced with permission.

Now as familiar superfoods continue to gain traction at even the largest national chains—turning once-obscure ingredients like kale, quinoa or açai into household names—some operators are looking to stand out by seeking lesser-known spices, seeds and produce that they expect to be part of the next wave of ultra-healthful ingredients.

Adding Appeal

There is no official definition for what makes a superfood, so the term has come to refer to almost any nutrient-packed item with purported health benefits. Current favorites on restaurant menus include fruits, such as blueberries or pomegranates; dark leafy greens, such as kale; ancients grains, like quinoa; and certain nuts, spices and seeds.

Superfoods generally make up only a small portion of menu items, but that's changing fast.

"They add sex appeal," said chef Matthew Kenney, who runs a raw-food culinary school in Santa Monica, Calif., and operates the adjacent M.A.K.E. restaurant and it's grab-and-go sister, M.A.K.E. Out. "The superfoods, in general, are really growing in popularity."

Marcus Antebi, the vegan, raw-foodist owner of Juice Press, a 10-unit chain in New York that sells hearty salads, nutrient-rich puddings and cold-pressed juices, said most of his customers recognize the inherent benefit of unprocessed fruits and vegetables, but noted that many guests still view superfoods as incredibly powerful and expect them to have a distinct positive impact on their health.

"[Customers seem to believe] there's some magical, mystical force in what I do at Juice Press, and they want to tap into that fountain of youth," he said.

Superfoods generally make up only a small portion of menu items, but that's changing fast. Kale and quinoa—two current poster children for healthful eating—make up just 2.9 percent and 1.9 percent of menus, respectively, according to research firm Datassential, but they've been showcased in recent rollouts from a number of chains.

For example, Gordon Biersch Brewery Restaurants has had a kale-quinoa pilaf on its menu for about three months at its 34 locations, and this month [April 2013] it rolled out a Superfood Salad with kale, blueberries, toasted smoked almonds, dried cranberries and feta cheese in lemon vinaigrette.

Breakfast-and-lunch chain First Watch has had a Quinoa Power Bowl with chicken, kale and roasted tomatoes on its menu since last winter, and Seasons 52, which called quinoa "grains of life" when it first put it on its vegetarian tasting menu last summer, now offers a quinoa salad with jicama, mint and cranberries.

Meanwhile, blueberries and pomegranate, two other prominent superfoods, will get some high-profile exposure when they're featured in a new addition to McDonald's Real Fruit Smoothies line in May.

Even as operators said these superfoods still have room to grow, some noted that these increasingly common superfoods are no longer enough to set a chain apart as a leader in healthful dining. In fact, some restaurants like Juice Press and M.A.K.E. that are on the front lines of the health-food trend say their customers already are seeking the next panacea.

"I've been watching all the trends, and there always seems to be a hot new item," said Alexis Schulze, chief visionary officer of 11-unit Nékter Juice Bar, based in Santa Ana, Calif.

Health-focused operators predicted the lesser-known products poised to become the next hot healthful items.

Turmeric

A potent root common in Indian curries, turmeric is believed to be a natural anti-inflammatory and is also high in antioxidants. It imparts a yellow color and mild bitterness when used in its dried form. When used fresh, it's an essential ingredient in many curries in southern Thailand, home of that country's spiciest food.

"I made a drink with turmeric a year ago," said Antebi of Juice Press. "It flopped. No one jumped on it. But I'm going to try again."

For that beverage, he combined the root, which he got fresh from Hawaii, with rose-infused water and orange juice.

Nékter's Schulze said making fresh turmeric palatable has been a challenge for her, too.

For audiences not ready for fresh turmeric, its cousin, ginger, may be an easier draw.

"It's got a really strong, harsh, almost cough-medicine-like flavor to it," she said.

But she has had success juicing it and adding it, along with another trendy superfood—cayenne pepper—to lemonade.

"It gives it an earthiness without that weird spicy bitterness," she said. "It's surprisingly refreshing."

Ginger

For audiences not ready for fresh turmeric, its cousin, ginger, may be an easier draw.

Another anti-inflammatory used to treat stomach ailments, fresh ginger is an established ingredient in trendy juice bars.

"Ginger is always an easy-selling item," Antebi of Juice Press said. "People feel warm and stimulated right off the bat."

Schulze puts fresh ginger in several of her juices at Nékter and also sells ginger shots made with an inch or two of juiced ginger, the juice of one lemon "and as much cayenne as people can handle," she said.

"It burns going down, but it relieves a lot of the discomfort associated with colds, sore throats and coughs," she said.

Katie Adair Barnhart, owner of Adair Kitchen in Houston, said her customers also respond well to ginger, which is a key ingredient in her Ginger Spice juice. That drink also contains spinach, carrot, green apple, celery and lemon.

Chia Seeds

Once known primarily in the context of the novelty items Chia Pets, this cousin of mint from southern Mexico and Guatemala also was a staple in the Aztec and Mayan diets, according to the website of wellness expert Dr. Andrew Weil. The seeds are also rich in omega-3 oils and fiber, according to Weil.

Weil's dietary principles, based on the anti-inflammatory properties of certain foods, are the basis for the menu at six-unit True Food Kitchen, a concept from Scottsdale, Ariz.-based Fox Restaurant Concepts.

True Food Kitchen offers a gluten-free, vegan chia-seed pudding, made with banana and coconut, on its dessert menu.

Similarly, Juice Press's Antebi makes a tapioca-like pudding out of chia seeds by soaking them in water for 30 minutes and adding cashew milk, which he makes by soaking raw cashews for between four and 10 hours then puréeing them for about four minutes. The dish is served cold.

Cashews

Nuts in general are good sources of antioxidants and mono-unsaturated fats, but John Inserra, executive vice president for restaurant operations and concept development for San Francisco-based Kimpton Hotel & Restaurant Group LLC, said cashews are a particularly popular component of the make-your-own trail-mix bars that were introduced as an option at catered events in March.

"It's kind of being listed as the go-to nut," he said.

Coconut

Kimpton also introduced smoothie bars as an option, and Inserra said juices were next. For both of those, he said, "coconut water is super important."

The cacao bean, the basis for chocolate, is appreciated for its antioxidants and is being added as a supplement to many juices in juice bars.

Kenney of M.A.K.E. agreed.

"Coconut, in general, is a really popular ingredient with our cuisine," he said, adding that one of M.A.K.E.'s most popular items is kimchi dumplings in a coconut-based wrapper.

Antebi said he adds coconut oil to Juice Press' truffles made from another trendy superfood: raw cacao.

Cacao

The cacao bean, the basis for chocolate, is appreciated for its antioxidants and is being added as a supplement to many juices in juice bars.

Kenney uses dried and fermented cacao rather than the more common roasted variety, tempering it with steam in a dehydrator at M.A.K.E.

"It's a little bit of a different take [from traditional chocolate], and it has a fermented taste to it, but it's delicious," he said, adding that he now prefers it to traditional chocolate.

"We make a lot of smoothies with raw cacao," said Antebi, who gets it in freeze-dried, powdered form at Juice Press. "And we put [it] in a few of our dessert dishes," he added.

Even more exotic superfoods may be on the way. Antebi's using more mangosteen—a tropical fruit popular in Southeast Asia and South Asia that's now cultivated in Hawaii. M.A.K.E.'s Kenney suggested that maqui berries from the Amazon might be the next goji berry. And both of them said they are using more maca, a Peruvian root with a malty flavor.

But in spite of the exotic new ingredients on the horizon, restaurants can never go wrong with simply offering a variety of fresh, unprocessed ingredients, Schulze of Nékter said.

"Fruits and vegetables, in general, are all superfoods," she said.

6

The Food Issue:
A Superfood Scientist Walks
Into a Farmers' Market

Mandy Oaklander

Mandy Oaklander is a former senior writer at Prevention.com, where she regularly covered health, science, and medicine.

Assigning the term superfood is not as simple as it might seem. Superfood rankings can't take into consideration so many compounds that haven't yet been measured or discovered. For produce shoppers, comparing the different nutritional benefits offered by fruits and vegetables, and making food choices depending on the health benefits you are seeking, is not easy. Thus, when selecting superfoods and other produce consumers should not rely solely on antioxidant claims or what is currently trendy.

Produce is trendy. Bradley Bolling is not. It's easy to spot him standing on the outskirts of Union Square Greenmarket in Manhattan—bespectacled with a crew cut, a plaid shirt tucked into belted khakis. This is fashion for a man most at home in a white coat and safety goggles. Bolling, 34, is a scientist, and his objects of study are the thousands of chemicals in the fruits and vegetables nestled inside all the reusable bags passing around us. You wouldn't know it from his unassuming vibe or his title (assistant professor in the department of nutritional sciences at the University of Connecticut), but he's

Mandy Oaklander, "The Food Issue: A Superfood Scientist Walks Into a Farmers' Market," *Prevention*, August 27, 2014. © 2014 Prevention. All rights reserved. Reproduced with permission.

famous among food scientists. Last year, after grinding up some almonds, Bolling and his students became the first group to discover a special class of tannins—a potential weapon against cancer and heart disease—in the nuts.

That kind of thing makes him a rock star to a nutrient hound like me, which is why I've asked him to shop for the produce at the very top of his personal superfood list, and then show me in his lab what superspecific powers he finds inside our purchases.

I'm not alone in my interest: Everyone here who gets wind of Bolling's pedigree clamors for usable nuggets. "What's the healthiest vegetable, Brad?" "Are raw-food diets better, Brad?" It's as if people are subjecting him to endless impromptu rounds of Trivial Pursuit: Vegetable Edition.

He tries to be enthusiastic. As a white-haired purveyor of ginger jelly waxes on about his fare, Bolling concurs gently, "Ginger has been studied for its antinausea effects."

Someone else asks him what the new kale should be. "Maybe Brussels sprouts?" Bolling answers.

Let's face it: We nonbiochemists cling to the healing promises of really long words—antioxidant, polyphenol, flavonoid, phytonutrient—without really getting what these terms mean or what science really knows about these substances.

You'd get about as many anthocyanins from one blueberry as you would if you ate a whole red apple.

Bolling knows, and it gives him pause. The pause is first apparent at the apple stand.

He holds in each hand an apple, one red, one green. "Really, the biggest difference is in the phytochemicals in the skin," he says. "Inside they're fairly similar." The red, he says, packs some anthocyanins, a type of flavonoid that gives red, purple, and blue produce their vivid hues and has been linked to lower levels of inflammation, better cognition, and reduced risks of cancer and Parkinson's disease.

"So you'd choose red over green?" I ask hopefully.

Bolling shrugs. "It probably doesn't make that big of a difference health-wise," he says. "You'd get about as many anthocyanins from one blueberry as you would if you ate a whole red apple."

So . . . forget both red and green apples and gorge on the blues?

Nope, not that, either, Bolling shrugs again. Apples are full of healthy fibers, acid, and other awesome compounds, he says, oblivious to my frustration.

There are reasons not to compare fruits or vegetables solely by their antioxidant reputations, he explains. Sure, antioxidants do the good work of binding with and neutralizing the free radicals that can cause inflammation and cell damage. But most aren't necessary for cell survival—and can actually damage proteins in our bodies. That's why our organs try to excrete many of them via natural enzyme systems. And why we have to consume them daily: to keep the nutrients around against our own bodies' volition.

This is a fact not lost on the purple-potato guy. As we cruise by his stand, a hot-orange sign catches our eyes: "THESE POTATOES HAVE EXTREMELY HIGH LEVELS OF ANTHOCYANINS—A POWERFUL ANTIOXIDANT!" it screams.

We pass by the bread stand, filled with loaves of nuts, seeds, and flax, which Bolling loves for their tocopherols (phytonutrients that include vitamin E), and then we reach the kale. It's deemed worthy of a purchase—thank God, since the number of kale salads I've suffered is too great for a scientist to declare it nutritionally mediocre. (Bolling identified some potently detoxifying compounds in kale 12 years ago, way before it ended up in the crispers of hipsters.)

We keep walking. I keep quizzing. Beets: They have to be good, given that last night he cooked them (sauteed and tossed with almond butter and hoisin) for his wife and two young sons, and he previously studied them for their anticarcinogenic activity. Herbs: A couple of bouquets go in the tote. A colleague, Bolling reports, is trying to isolate the antimicrobial compounds of thyme to feed it to animals and possibly cut the antibiotic load farmers feed chickens. "Herbs and spices are some of the richest sources of polyphenols in a diet, but we typically don't eat enough of them to have that big of an impact," he says.

With that, he steers me toward the jam stand. I'm surprised—after all the caveats about ranking superfoods, sugar is cool with the food scientist?

"It's a good way to keep your berries," he says, and to preserve the antioxidants along with them. Turns out we've finally hit on Bolling's main scientific squeeze: He studies (and makes his own jam from) aronia berries, aka chokeberries. These beauties are loaded with anthocyanins, he says—you can tell because they're almost black. In his work, Bolling is looking into how the aronia berry may ease inflammatory bowel disease, lower cholesterol, and reduce inflammation. Right now, though, he's looking into jam jars and coming up short: no aronias. We settle on a blueberry-ginger preserve instead.

We don't have enough information to say definitively that a tomato is better than a cucumber.

At this point, I'm at my wit's end. C'mon, Brad, if all these plant chemicals act like pharmaceuticals in our bodies, helping to prevent or ease chronic disease, which ones do we want, and how much of them do we need?

"People are always trying to create these superfoods and superfood rankings," he finally says. "But there are so many compounds we haven't measured that are not included in those rankings—probably hundreds, if not thousands, of undiscovered plant compounds."

In other words, we don't have enough information to say definitively that a tomato is better than a cucumber.

"Who knows?" he says. "There might be something awesome in cucumbers that nobody's looked for yet."

A week later, strapped into plastic goggles and a white coat at Bolling's lab, I'm the one who looks like a nerd. He's in his element. He flits among the filing cabinets filled with beakers of all sizes, prepping for our experiment. We won't be discovering any unknown supercompounds, but we will tease out known anthocyanins, carotenoids, and other antioxidants that hide within our farmers' market bounty, mashing it all up to extract the pigments.

I dump our haul on the counter.

"Is this all the kale you have?" Bolling asks, eyeing a few wrinkly stalks.

"Yeah," I say. "I ate the rest of it for dinner last night."

"Well, at least you got the nutrients."

Bolling's plan is to show me the pigment-extraction process known as chromatography. We'll blend the fruits and vegetables with alcohol, then separate the pigmented anthocyanins and carotenoids from the rest of the mix so we can see their pure concentrations. It's the first step for anything that Bolling studies quantitatively, from the chemicals in pure fruits and vegetables to those same nutrients in human blood or mouse intestines after digestion. A question he and his team are trying to answer: If your blood shows a greater concentration of a phytonutrient than the next person's after you both eat the same amount of something like aronia berries, might you have more protection against heart disease?

Spoiler alert: We have no idea. Again. Science has figured out face transplants, but we still don't know precisely what's in a berry or what exactly happens when you eat it.

Chromatography is everyday stuff for Bolling, but the implications of this type of research for the future of medicine are huge. By measuring someone's phytonutrient levels, scientists could one day tailor recommendations to restore the nutrients that the person lacks or excretes more readily than other people do. "I think with enough research, we can get down to the level of recommending individual foods for individual conditions or specific chronic diseases," Bolling says.

He hacks into a tomato with a pair of box cutters, and guts spurt from its tomato warts. "This smells good—too bad we can't eat it," he murmurs. A knife would have worked better, but Bolling is moving to the University of Wisconsin next week to start a new job as an assistant professor, and it's packed in a box somewhere. He throws each bludgeoned piece of food into a beaker, adds some alcohol—"A little smoothie!"—and whirs it all with a hand blender.

After all the fruit cocktails are prepared, Bolling pours the liquid into test tubes and flips on the extraction vacuum. Bands of vivid greens and pinks and oranges emerge like sand art in bottles at a county fair. We huddle over the rainbow-ringed test tubes. "So those are the extracted anthocyanins?" I ask, peering at the pretty pink bands in the test tube full of macerated beets.

"Yeah, this is the purified pigment here in the betalains," he says, referring to the substance found in beets and some flower petals.

Because dietary studies are expensive and sometimes unethical to do on humans, [scientists] often feed mice a ton of fruit or nuts to find out how the polyphenols are distributed in the rodents' livers, brains, and intestines.

"I guess you could just drink those."

You can't, of course, because the alcohol we added would poison you, Bolling corrects me. But you could neutralize the acid and end up with the purified anthocyanins that are used as colorants for different products. This is how companies put the lip-staining red in slushies or the fruit or vegetable extract in supplements.

One thing we're missing is Bolling's fave, the aronia berry. Luckily, this lab appears to be the aronia capital of Connecticut. On our way to gather some from the freezers, we pass unfortunate students extracting guinea-pig eyeballs in the pitch dark (eyeball extraction is light-sensitive work, Bolling tells me), blending them up (yum), and measuring how much dietary lutein makes it into the peepers. When I ask about the nearby freezer that reads "Call Rick when the freezer is full," Bolling explains, "Oh, there are a bunch of dead mice and animal carcasses in there. Rick never really answers."

We finally find a bag of frozen aronia berries in another freezer, wedged next to a box full of vials marked "fetal bovine serum" (great for growing human cells, by the way). Because dietary studies are expensive and sometimes unethical to do on humans, Bolling and his team often feed mice a ton of fruit or nuts to find out how the polyphenols are distributed in the rodents' livers, brains, and intestines.

Back in his lab, Bolling decants the harvest into a beaker. I ask for a taste, but he makes me take a berry from a freezer for people food instead. I pop it into my mouth. It's the sourest thing in the world. I don't care how many antioxidants are in them—nobody would eat these raw.

"I have them almost every day on my oatmeal," Bolling tells me. I scrunch up my face at the thought. "Or if you just bake them into an apple crisp," he concedes, "that's good, too."

There! Even while trying to understand how we absorb plant compounds and what powers certain foods have, Bolling is committed to eating like a superfood superfan. Like me.

As for the science, he's currently pitting aronia berries against mouse colitis. Despite what my taste buds tell me, I'm betting on the berries.

7

Kale Is a Superfood

Sayer Ji

Sayer Ji is founder and director of GreenMedInfo.com and an advisory board member of the nonprofit National Health Federation.

As a superfood, kale is essentially unrivaled in nutritional density. With a 3:1 carbohydrate-to-protein ratio, the form of cabbage possesses an exceptional amount of protein for a vegetable, which is why it's the "new beef." In fact, like meat, kale contains all nine essential amino acids needed in the formation of proteins in the human body in addition to nine nonessential amino acids. It contains more omega-3 than omega-6, making it an anomaly of nature. Kale is also the new "vegetable cow." Compared to whole milk, it has more calcium per gram and is better absorbed in the body. Last but not least, biomedical research shows that the leafy green may be useful in treating cancer, glaucoma, and other conditions.

Few foods commonly available at the produce stand are as beneficial to your health as kale. And yet, sadly, it is more commonly found dressing up something not as healthy in a display case as a decoration than on someone's plate where it belongs.

Kale is actually a form of cabbage that evaded domestication, sharing many of the same traits as wilder plant relatives unafraid of holding on to their bitter principle, and relatively unruly appearance.

Kale is perfectly content letting its luscious green leafy hair down, being the 'hippie' member of a family that includes the more tightly wound broccoli, cauliflower and the Brussels sprout, whose greater respectability is as far as most restaurant menus go.

This means kale is more likely to be found forgotten, shriveling up somewhere on the bottom shelf of someone's refrigerator, no doubt possessed by someone with every intention (but not the time and appetite enough) to eat it.

But please do not underestimate this formidable plant, which grows as high as six to seven feet in the right conditions, casting a shadow as long as the impressive list of beneficial nutritional components it contains.

Indeed, like meat, kale contains all 9 essential amino acids needed to form the proteins within the human body.

Its nutritional density, in fact, is virtually unparalleled among green leafy vegetables. Consider too that during World War II, with rationing in full effect, the U.K. [United Kingdom] encouraged the backyard cultivation of this hearty, easy to grow plant for the *Dig for Victory* campaign that likely saved many from sickness and starvation. Over a half century later, kale's status as a former cultural nutritional hero has faded into near oblivion . . . until now, we hope!

Kale Contains ALL the Essential Amino Acids and 9 Non-Essential Ones

You will notice that one cup of raw kale contains less than 1 gram of fat (0.3 grams to be exact), 2 grams of protein, and subtracting the 1 gram of fiber from the total carbohydrate content (7), an effective carb content of 6 grams per serving, which is almost entirely complex carbohydrate, i.e. "starch." This means it has a 3:1 carbohydrate-to-protein ratio—an exceptionally high amount of protein for any vegetable, and one reason why it has recently been acclaimed as the "new beef."

Indeed, like meat, kale contains all 9 essential amino acids needed to form the proteins within the human body: histidine, isoleucine, leucine, lysine, methionine, phenylalanine, threonine, tryptophan, valine—plus, 9 other non-essential ones for a total of 18.

Consider too that compared to meat, the amino acids in kale are easier to extract. When consuming a steak, for instance, the body has to expend great metabolic resources to break down the massive, highly complex, and intricately folded protein structures within mammalian flesh back down into their constituent amino acids.

Then, later, these extracted amino acids must be reassembled back into the same, highly complex, intricately folded and refolded human proteins from which our body is made. This is a time-consuming, energy-intensive process, with many metabolic waste products released in the process.

For the same reason that massive mammalian herbivores like cows, for instance, eat grass—not other animals—kale can be considered anabolic, "meaty," and worthy of being considered as a main course in any meal. The nice thing, too, is that less is needed to fulfill the body's protein requirements.

Also, kale is so much lower on the food chain than beef, that it doesn't bio-accumulate as many, and as much, of the toxins in our increasingly polluted environment. And this, of course, doesn't even touch on the great "moral debate" concerning avoiding unnecessary harm to sentient beings, i.e. eating kale is morally superior than eating/killing animals.

Kale Is an Omega-3 Diamond in the Rough

While it is considered a "fat-free" vegetable, it does contain biologically significant quantities of essential fatty acids—you know, the ones your body is not designed to create and *must* get from the things we eat or suffer dire consequences.

In fact, you will notice it contains *more* omega-3 than omega-6, which is almost unheard of in nature. It is a general rule that you will find a 40:1 or higher ratio of omega-6 to omega-3 found in most grains, seeds, nuts and beans. Peanuts, for instance, have 1,800 times higher omega-6 fat levels than omega-3, which (taken in isolation) is a pro-inflammatory and unhealthy ratio. Kale, therefore, is a superstar as far as essential fatty acids go, and especially considering that all of its naturally-occurring fat-soluble antioxidants protect these fragile unsaturated fats from oxidizing.

Those who know kale well, can feel a happy little glow form within them after consuming it.

Kale's Vitamin Content Pays for Itself Many Times Over

Now to the vitamins. Kale is a king of carotenoids. Its vitamin A activity is astounding. One cup contains over 10,000 IUs, or the equivalent of over 200% the daily value. Also, consider that most of this vitamin A (retinol) is delivered in the form of beta-carotene, which in its natural form is the perfect delivery system for retinol (two retinol molecules attached to one another), as it is exceedingly difficult to get too much. If you compare it to the synthetic vitamin A used in many mass market foods and vitamins, it is an order of magnitude or higher safer.

Kale Is an Eye-Saving Superfood Rich in Vitamins

Kale has a few more surprises left in the "vitamin" department. It turns out that it is loaded with both lutein and zeaxanthin at over 26 mg combined, per serving. Lutein comes from the Latin word luteus meaning "yellow," and is one of the best known carotenoids in a family containing at least

600. In the human eye, it is concentrated in the retina in an oval-shaped yellow spot near its center known as the macula (from Latin *macula*, "spot" + *lutea*, "yellow"). This "yellow spot" acts as a natural sunblock, which is why adequate consumption of lutein and zeaxanthin may prevent macular degeneration and other retinal diseases associated with ultraviolet light-induced oxidative stress.

Keep in mind that a 26 mg dose of lutein + zeaxanthin can easily cost $1 per dose. In effect, one could calculate the cost reduction of this added bonus into kale's sticker price, which incidentally, is insultingly low considering all it has to offer. How, after all, does one price the preservation of your vision?

Next, the vitamin C content, at over 80 mg per serving, is impressive. Consider, this is not ascorbic acid (which is semi-synthetic, and divorced from the food factors that help confer its amazing vitamin activity). Food vitamin C is a rare and precious element in the modern diet that is an absolute requirement for us to maintain our health. It can be likened to condensed sunlight frozen within the plant and released into our bodies after we eat it. Those who know kale well, can feel a happy little glow form within them after consuming it. And, I imagine, if we had the proper measuring device, we might see a slight uptick in intensity of the biophotons that are continually emitted from our body.

Kale: The New "Vegetable Cow"?

Now, just when you thought kale was just too good to be true, there is the matter of its remarkable mineral composition. Of course, the quality and mineral and microbial density of the soil within which it is grown is a factor, but kale generally has the ability to provide an excellent source of minerals, in what is known as food-state. Unlike inorganic minerals, e.g. limestone, bone meal, oyster shell, the calcium in kale is vibrating with life-sustaining energy and intelligence.

At 90 milligrams per cup, this highly bioavailable calcium actually contains more calcium per gram than whole milk! Also, a calcium bioavailability study from 1990, comparing milk and kale in human subjects, found that kale calcium was 25% better absorbed, proving that the propaganda in support of milk as the ultimate source of calcium isn't as mooo-ving as commonly believed.

Just to be a bit exact about how much calcium there is in kale, for every gram of kale there is 1.35 mg of calcium. For every gram of whole milk, there is 1.13 mg. The difference, also, is that milk calcium is complexed with a sticky protein known as casein. This is why Elmer's glue was once made of milk protein. It is exceedingly hard for one-stomached (monogastric) mammals (that's us) to digest, and so, the calcium is difficult, if not impossible (in some) to liberate.

Kale is more than just a nutritional "superfood." . . . *Newly emergent biomedical literature now shows it may be of value in the treatment of cancer, elevated blood lipids, glaucoma, and various forms of chemical poisoning.*

Also, casein proteins require a large amount of hydrochloric acid to break down with our protein-digesting pancreatic enzymes. Over time, this can lead to some metabolic acidosis which may further leach calcium from our mineral stores.

For example, bones [and] teeth, causing a net loss in calcium following the consumption of cow's milk products heavy in casein, especially cheese. Kale, like most vegetables, on the other hand, are alkalinizing and therefore actually reduce the body's requirements for acid-neutralizing minerals (e.g. calcium, magnesium, sodium, silica, potassium) and therefore reducing the total amount of calcium we need to stay in pH and mineral balance. Kale, therefore, not only contains more of the *right form* of calcium, but may actually reduce your daily bodily requirements for it. Move over moo juice, there's a new "vegetable cow" on the block!

Kale is also an excellent source of magnesium, *which is why it is green*. That deep, dark chlorophyll within its leaves contains one atom of magnesium per molecule. And considering how many of us are dying from excess elemental calcium, adding additional sources of magnesium (which acts to balance out calcium) can have life-saving health benefits.

Finally, kale is more than just a nutritional "superfood." It comes from a long line of plant healers, and could very well be considered and (given future FDA [Food and Drug Administration] drug approval) used as a medicine. Newly emergent biomedical literature now shows it may be of value in the treatment of cancer, elevated blood lipids, glaucoma, and various forms of chemical poisoning.

We have made available the first-hand abstracts on our Kale Health Benefits research page, for those who, like us, enjoy geeking out to the science. Also, kale, like most cruciferous vegetables, is exceedingly high in several other extensively researched anticancer compounds, such as sulforaphane and indole-3-carbinol. The data set on these are even more impressive than on kale itself, with over 140 disease states potential remedies for sulforaphane alone.

8

Increasing Quinoa Production Has Harmful Environmental Impacts

Mark Hawthorne

Mark Hawthorne is a writer, animal activist, and vegan. He is author of Bleating Hearts: The Hidden World of Animal Suffering *and* Striking at the Roots: A Practical Guide to Animal Activism.

While quinoa is now hailed as a miracle food and is gaining worldwide interest, production of the commodity in Bolivia and Peru, where 92 percent of the grain is grown, is causing negative environmental impacts and changing traditional farming practices. To keep up with demand, the most vulnerable farmers now work year-round, depleting the soil they rely on to survive and maintain their culture. Also, industrialized farming and global warming are bringing pests to previously unaffected regions, leading to the use of pesticides and agrochemicals. And making way for more quinoa crops moves grazing llamas, which help prevent erosion, off these lands. To support Bolivia and Peru, the most conscientious choice for consumers is to buy organic, fair trade-certified quinoa.

Today, quinoa—with its off-the-charts nutritional value—is hailed as nothing short of a miracle food and is granted a primo position on supermarket shelves. The United Nations declared 2013 the International Year of Quinoa. Not bad for a humble crop that is cultivated almost exclusively in the Andes Mountains. But lately, quinoa has gone from superfood to serious food for thought. Critics contend that since quinoa became a foodie favorite in the west several years ago, the Andean staple has tripled in price, resulting in land disputes, a collapse of traditional farming practices, and unhealthy diet changes in Bolivia and Peru, which together account for 92 percent of the world's production.

The controversy has been simmering for a couple of years, but it was brought to a rapid boil in January [2013] with a piece in *The Guardian* that left more than a few ethical eaters hot and bothered. The article "Can Vegans Stomach the Unpalatable Truth about Quinoa?" chided herbivores about devouring the plant-powered food and was suspiciously light on outside sources. The *Globe and Mail* followed, declaring succinctly, "The more you love quinoa, the more you hurt Peruvians and Bolivians." Soon the biogosphere was all atwitter with reproachful posts, and conscientious consumers were left wondering what to make of it all. So, who's right? Are ethical eaters hurting humans with their appetite for quinoa, or are ethical producers ensuring a fortuitous future for Bolivians by cultivating the crop?

Bolivians in general do not eat much quinoa, and it's been that way for 500 years.

Ancient Harvest

For Andean farmers, "the mother grain" was not only an essential food but part of their religious ceremonies and burial rituals. Each year, it was the Incan emperor who broke the soil with a golden spade and planted the first seed. But Spanish conquistadors, who arrived in Peru in 1531, scorned quinoa and forbade its cultivation under penalty of death. They forced the natives to replace their ancestral crops with European species such as wheat and barley, and quinoa's popularity waned. It continued to flourish in the wild, however, and as the South American colonies fought for and gradually gained their independence from Spain during the 19th century, quinoa was poised to be rediscovered and reintroduced.

Myth-Busting

The nascent quinoa craze, coupled with the international market's potential for dramatic worldwide consequences, does have experts concerned, but not that Bolivians can no longer afford to eat the stuff. "That's one of the very compelling myths," says Tanya Kerssen, analyst for the Oakland [California]-based think tank Food First, which works to end injustices that cause world hunger. "The quinoa producers eat quinoa. They reserve part of their harvest for home consumption, I think sometimes they'll buy less-nutritious rice and bread and pasta—that's true across the board; it's not just quinoa farmers who do that. Also, they get sick of eating quinoa, frankly, so they buy other foods." Filmmakers Michael Wilcox and Stefan Jeremiah saw that firsthand when they met with Bolivian farmers for their upcoming documentary *The Mother Grain*, which explores the effects of quinoa's growing popularity. "Just like you and I might not want to eat quinoa every day, they might not want to eat quinoa every day," says Wilcox. Inspired by all the recent attention focused on quinoa, the filmmakers initially went to the Andes to photograph the harvest, hoping to produce a coffee-table book. "But when we started speaking to people and doing research, we found this story. They are earning more money to invest back into their communities and their farms to grow better-quality quinoa than they ever have before to meet with the rising global demand."

Also speaking from experience is Sergio Nuñez de Arco, a quinoa specialist with US importer Andean Naturals, who adds that quinoa is not even really a staple in Bolivia. "That's another myth," he says. "I was born and raised in Bolivia, and I never ate quinoa. Never. Nor did my friends. Bolivians in general do not eat much quinoa, and it's been that way for 500 years." It's the farmers who eat most of the quinoa, he says, and lots of it. "As the market prices have gone up and demand has increased, they have grown more. So whereas they used to consume 80 percent of what they grew, now they probably consume 10 percent." Nuñez de Arco adds that stories of land disputes have little or nothing to do with quinoa. "There are violent conflicts over land, but there have been violent conflicts over land in the Andes for a thousand years." The international development organization Mercy Corps reports that up to 70 percent of farmable land in Bolivia is held by only a few thousand large landowners, and 65 percent of the population lives below the poverty line. It's not difficult to imagine why disenfranchised indigenous farmers—unable to prove a parcel of land that's been in their family for generations is legally theirs—would aggressively attempt to assert their rights.

The problem [with quinoa], it turns out, is not really dietary but environmental.

Looking beyond the misinformation, it seems clear that the global enthusiasm for quinoa has largely been beneficial. "I think the quinoa boom has been good in general for Bolivia and Bolivians," says Emma Banks of the Andean Information Network, an NGO [nongovernmental organization] promoting human rights and socioeconomic justice. As Banks points out, they're eating more than ever. "Over the last five years, quinoa consumption in Bolivia has actually tripled."

This increase in consumption comes even as prices have gone up, though what most reports overlook is that basic salaries have also risen in Bolivia. Last year [in 2012], the government implemented an 8 percent increase in the minimum wage, and Bolivian President Evo Morales facilitated a $10 million loan for farmers to grow more quinoa. Morales, a former quinoa farmer himself, was named Special Ambassador for the International Year of Quinoa, along with Peru's first lady, Nadine Heredia, both of whom advocate for better nutrition for mothers and children. "That is why the government of Bolivia is supplying quinoa as part of a nutritional supplement program to pregnant and nursing women, and Peru is incorporating quinoa in school breakfasts," said UN [United Nations] Secretary-General Ban Ki-moon at the launch of the International Year of Quinoa in February.

The Dirt on Quinoa

The problem, it turns out, is not really dietary but environmental. Kerssen notes that the potential desertification of the growing region should also be factored into consideration. She believes turning this sacred seed from a subsistence crop into a prized commodity is leading the poorest, most vulnerable farmers to work the soil year-round, degrading the very land they depend on for survival and cultural identity. Among the Andean ecological disruptions keeping Kerssen awake at night are the effects of mechanized soil tilling, one of the hallmarks of industrialized agriculture. "When you combine that with global warming and higher temperatures in that region, you've got the perfect recipe for greater incidence of pests," she says. In a region where pesticides are practically unheard of—bugs are rare above 12,000 feet—insects are beginning to appear, leading some farmers to use insecticides and other agrochemicals to maintain production. And of course, once farmers begin using pesticides, they eliminate not only the bugs they are targeting but also the helpful critters. As a result, one of quinoa's fundamental appeals—its organic status—could be compromised.

Exacerbating the environmental dilemma is that the llamas who once grazed and fertilized traditional farms—and helped prevent erosion with their large, padded feet—are being moved off the land to make way for more quinoa crops. Sven-Erik Jacobsen, associate professor of plant and environmental sciences at the University of Copenhagen in Denmark, believes that the environmental consequences include an overall decline in crop yield. "However, it does not need to have these effects, but the right measures have to be taken to counteract them." One solution Jacobsen proposes is to grow quinoa in other countries yet maintain a high-value product for export in Bolivia. For example, he notes that the type of quinoa known as Real (or Royal) is adapted to the specific conditions in southern Bolivia, with the region's extreme drought and saline-infused soils. But other types of quinoa can easily flourish elsewhere, such as in Africa, where Jacobsen is working to grow it.

Andean quinoa has a bushel full of defenders, who see [US] production as a threat to the people of South America's Altipiano.

Cultivating the Future

Although Jacobsen is confident he can help bring quinoa to the masses by producing it well beyond the shadow of the Andes, others aren't so sure that's the solution. Ernie New began growing quinoa in the Colorado Rocky Mountains in 1984, and while his White Mountain Farm is flush with potatoes and other organic veggies, the mother grain has been less than nurturing. "We're not able to grow much," he says. "Most of the time our supply is gone long before the demand has dried up." Cultivation experiments in Africa may prove successful, but New doesn't believe quinoa is a viable crop in the United States. "It does well in some climates, but it is susceptible to wind and heat. You're not going to get people to plow the ski slopes of Colorado to grow quinoa."

New's experience is discouraging, especially considering that his was the first large-scale quinoa operation in the country. White Mountain Farm planted 120 acres of quinoa last year, yet they were able to harvest only 70 after a harsh summer. "If it gets above 90 degrees during the flowering stage, it won't produce seeds," New explains.

But the USDA [US Department of Agriculture] is backing quinoa, and recently awarded a $1.6 million grant to Washington State University researchers, who will spend the next three years conducting an extensive trial to identify the varieties best suited for organic production. "I do believe that quinoa can be grown commercially in this area, but there are several hurdles that we and growers face," says Kevin Murphy, lead scientist and plant breeder for the project. "For example, selection of varieties for early maturity is important, as is resistance to downy mildew and pre-harvest sprouting." The trials have been promising, and Murphy reports there's a lot of interest from farmers, distributors, and retailers for Washington-grown quinoa.

Andean quinoa has a bushel full of defenders, who see domestic production as a threat to the people of South America's Altipiano, the mountain plateau where the perfect blend of altitude, climate, and soil has made it the world's quinoa basket. "Growing quinoa in North America only takes the market away from quinoa farmers in Bolivia and Peru," says Banks. "The Altipiano is historically incredibly poor with few resources. Quinoa is one of the only means of income for people who live there." Wilcox shares the sentiment, adding, "I've seen comments on some of these anti-quinoa articles, like, 'Thanks for shining a light on the truth. I won't consume Bolivian quinoa because it's hurting these farmers.' Well, not consuming it is really going to hurt these farmers. They'll be stuck with a dry pile of quinoa and no income to support their families."

Perhaps the most effective way for conscientious consumers to support Bolivia and Peru is to buy organic quinoa that is certified Fair Trade. Doing so helps farmers and their families earn better wages for their hard work, allowing them to keep their children in school, hold on to their land, preserve their cultural heritage, and invest in the quality and productivity of their harvest. "Most consumers just care about price," says Nuñez de Arco. "Consumers have the power to generate a demand that creates an alignment of the whole supply chain. If they go to Trader Joe's and ask, 'Is this bag of Bolivian quinoa fairly traded? Am I part of something that's not good?' All of a sudden, Trader Joe's calls us and says, 'Tell me again about that Fair Trade thing. What do we have to do? Ten cents more? Sure, just do it.'"

The saga of quinoa is closely tied to food security and sovereignty, and it's one that should ultimately be written by active citizens, not passive consumers. Whether quinoa retains its organic roots and benefits farmers and customers alike or becomes a genetically modified global commodity monopolized by socially irresponsible corporations is really up to us.

9

Edible Insects Are the Next Superfood

Jahred Liddie

Jahred Liddie is a student at Harvard University and managing editor of the Harvard College Review of Environment and Society.

Edible insects have been ignored as a sustainable superfood in much of the world. Crickets, for example, are high in protein but low in fat compared to beef. Furthermore, making food with them can significantly reduce water usage, demands for feed, and greenhouse gas emissions; in fact, crickets can be raised in small spaces and urban areas, closing the distance between farm and table. However, because of deeply negative reactions in the United States, many people still refuse to eat them. Young entrepreneurs hope to change attitudes and make "entotarian," a person who eats insects and no other meat, a household name.

I recently had the opportunity to interview Rose Wang and Laura D'Asaro on their innovative startup, Six Foods. Along with Meryl Natow, the Harvard College graduates of the Class of 2013 are on a mission to create a buzz in the food industry ... with crickets. Yes, you read that correctly: Six Foods incorporates bugs, such as crickets, into its products. Housed in the Harvard Innovation Labs's new Launch Lab space, Six Foods currently boasts a selection of "chirps"—chips made with cricket flour—and holiday cricket cookies. Both products are made with cricket flour, a nutty flour of roasted and milled crickets. A chirp, gluten-free and baked, has three times the protein and half the fat of a normal potato chip. Just in time for the holiday season, the chocolate chip cricket cookie, with a hint of cinnamon, has five grams of protein per serving.

The entrepreneurs were as eager to talk as I was to be at the Launch Lab—an energetic space, alive with the quickened pace of start-ups of all kinds. They greeted me with smiles, chit chat, and, of course, a basket full of holiday cookies. Had I been given these cookies in any other context, I would have assumed they were regular old homemade cookies that your grandmother could have made—but these cookies were made with a special, secret ingredient. High in crickets and in flavor, Six Foods' products are *not* your grandmother's cookies; they challenge their non-bug counterparts, and ask us why we eat the way that we do.

Crickets are dense in protein but light in fat relative to their beef counterparts, but there is a list of other pros that these insects present.

A Miracle Food Ignored

Laura was first introduced to insects as food in her under-graduate years on a trip to Africa, around the same time when Rose returned from a trip to China. Laura ate caterpillars in Tanzania, and was fascinated with how entrenched insects were into the local culture. In another area of the world, a friend dared Rose to eat a scorpion. It tasted just like shrimp, due to the close evolutionary ties between the two organisms.

The two former students began doing their research once they were together again on campus, and began sampling reci-pes with friends. What started out as just fun became more of a business, and the three students entered a startup competition with tacos made with mealworms as their entry. Soon after, Six Foods was launched.

As you may have gleaned, crickets are dense in protein but light in fat relative to their beef counterparts, but there is a list of other pros that these insects present. Elaborating on this subject, Laura first envisioned the future we're heading towards: a larger world population means a larger demand for water and food. With food made from insects, we can reduce water usage, feed demands, and greenhouse gas emissions by several magnitudes. Additionally, 1000 crickets can survive in a small space, even in urban areas, reducing the distance from farm to table. Rose continued that this could create a more closed-loop food system, and could engage city residents in "urban farming," a particularly weighty point, given that more and more will move to cities. "It seems like this [is a] miracle food that everyone had ignored," she stated.

But if insects are miracle foods, why aren't they in our refrigerators right now? Rose, a former Psychology concentrator, observed that friends who sampled test goods displayed either deeply positive or negative reactions, which helped to drum up a lot of attention. She elaborated that many in the United States think that, as citizens of a developed country, they should not have to resort to insects. Investing in the future with their products, Six Foods aims to change minds, and uses a concerted meld of social media and education to disperse information swiftly in this information age. Next, Laura added that Americans object to eating whole version of things that they already eat, a wasteful convention that insects would remove. She reflected that a non-native professor, who had eaten grasshoppers but had never had shrimp, thought of shrimp as just "sea grasshoppers." Conversely, Six Foods wants to familiarize insects with the food culture of the United States.

Enter the "Entotarian"

Lastly, the two ruminated on their current progress and future goals for Six Foods. With the recent launch, both are excited to see their product on the shelf and meet someone who has heard of their foods indirectly—symbols and milestones of all of the effort and difficulties in popularizing insects as food. At some point, Laura envisions that the company will release products with insects as a meat form, further reducing the environmental impacts of our calories. She wants "entotarian," a person whose diet includes insects and no other meats, to become a household phrase. I was excited for them too, for these short-term goals and for their foray to leave a mark on our changing food web in the future. Giving closure to these big dreams, Rose remarked, "It's about taking these ingredients on a journey, basically the same journeys we went though."

10

Juicing Can Benefit Health

Lisa Sussman

Lisa Sussman is author of several books on health and nutrition, including Cold Press Juice Bible: 300 Delicious, Nutritious, All-Natural Recipes for Your Masticating Juicer.

More than two-thirds of adults do not eat the recommended daily servings of fruits and vegetables. Enter juicing. It squeezes pounds' worth of produce high in vitamins, minerals, and anti-oxidants into a single glass, making it easier and tastier to consume. But it must be at-home juicing: buying them at juice bars is very expensive, and bottled brands lack freshly squeezed nutrients and may have additives. Cold-press juicing is best—it slowly presses the produce with less oxygen, heat, and pulp along with more liquid. However, juices should have a 4:1 ratio of vegetables to fruit to ensure a low, healthy amount of sugar.

Fact: You're not eating enough vegetables and fruit. It doesn't matter if you're working up a daily sweat trying to add more crops to your diet. You could be doing everything from throwing bushels of blueberries into your morning cereal to turning your grab-a-cheese-pizza-on-the-way-home into a veritable salad bar buffet of toppings; chances are that you, like more than two-thirds of adults, aren't hitting the USDA [US Department of Agriculture] target of nine servings of produce every day (translation: four half-cup servings of fruit and five half-cup servings of vegetables). These are not grandiose goals here. Many nutrition experts would argue that nine servings a day of fruits and vegetables is the bare minimum.

What you're missing out on could make all the difference between fizzling and sizzling health-wise. It seems we really are what we eat. Diets stuffed with fruits and vegetables not only have a heavy impact on weight management, they also reduce risk on some of the leading causes of death. According to studies from Johns Hopkins University, all it takes is one apple a day—or a peach or 10 baby carrots or a half-cup of whipped rutabaga—to lower heart disease risk by 20 percent. The Harvard School of Public Health prescribes a high dose of vegetables and fruits to help lower blood pressure, reduce the risk of cardiac disease and stroke, prevent some types of cancer, lessen the risk of eye and digestive problems, and help to lower blood sugar (the last of which, in turn, will help keep appetite in check).

With juice, you're literally squeezing a couple of pounds of vitamin-, mineral- and antioxidant-rich produce into a glass.

In nutritional terms, vegetables especially, but also fruits, are pretty near the perfect food: low in fat and loaded with a myriad of important vitamins, minerals and antioxidants that fight all kinds of illnesses. As a study published in the *American Journal of Epidemiology* concludes, those daily nine servings, especially when eaten raw, will reduce your risk of death by as much as 10 percent and, for every extra three helpings, drop risk by another 6 percent. And, under the "It's Not Fair" heading, the benefits are even higher for those still struggling with their New Year's resolutions: When they pile on the produce, drinkers can soak up to a 40 percent mortality reduction, the obese weigh in with a 20 percent mortality reduction and there's even some evidence that smokers may also inhale some benefits. Researchers conjecture that these higher rewards may be due to antioxidants strutting their stuff which, in turn, takes the edge off the oxidative stress caused by many of these bad habits.

So the big debate isn't whether you need more fruit and vegetables in your life—you do. The question is, how you are going to get those vegetables and fruit into your body.

Hello, juice! Granted, eating vegetables in their whole form is usually the best answer. However, chomping through half of a grapefruit, a half-cup of strawberries, an apple, a banana, a cup of spinach, a half-cup of carrots, a half-cup of red peppers, a handful of asparagus stalks and a half-cup of green beans (for example) every single day can seem like the definition of impossible unless you're part groundhog. But with juice, you're literally squeezing a couple of pounds of vitamin-, mineral- and antioxidant-rich produce into a glass, which is going to be both easier and tastier to chug down.

Plus, these drinks, especially when homemade, are automatically low in the ingredients blacklisted by doctors and nutritionists. These include fats, processed sugars, artificial anything and salt. While the jury is still out on whether your body can absorb the nutrients more easily in liquid form or if there's any advantage in giving your digestive system a break from working on fiber, there is sound evidence that drinking juice delivers the goodness, and most nutrient-dense part of the food, in a concentrated form. A US Department of Agriculture study found that 90 percent of the antioxidant activity, especially cancer-fighting carotenoids (which are found in carrots, spinach, apricots, tomatoes and red bell peppers, to name a few), is in the juice rather than the fiber. The *American Journal of Medicine* concluded in a study that people who quaffed 3+ servings per week of juices high in polyphenols (antioxidants found in purple grape, grapefruit, cranberry and apple juice) had a 76 percent lower risk of developing Alzheimer's disease.

The fact that the fruits and vegetables are eaten raw means that in some cases, you ingest even more of those super nutrients. . . . In short, even the most expensive vitamin pill can't begin to match the nutritional complexity of a fresh juice.

Not Your Bottled Brand

This juice isn't your morning gulp of Florida fresh. This juice is also a verb—juicing is the process of extracting juices from fresh fruits and vegetables using machines specifically designed to (depending on the style) either pulverize, crush or blend the produce to make a fresh and unpasteurized liquid that contains most of the vitamins, minerals and plant chemicals (phytonutrients) found in the whole fruit.

Buying a juicer is like purchasing a home—you're investing for the long-term.

One reason juice has become a must-have for all that is good for you is that these machines are now available for home use. And although it sometimes seems like you can't throw an avocado pit these days without hitting a juice bar or a store stocked with every kind of juice from acai to zesty beet, it turns out that it pays to play [lifestyle expert] Martha Stewart and juice it yourself.

While the fare at juice bars is more like homemade, it comes with the kind of sticker price usually associated with top-shelf cocktails because you're not only paying for the produce, you're subsidizing the bar's commercial version of the appliance, their real estate lease, the salaries of the workers, the monthly utility fees, the store's pet mascot and so on. In short, when it comes to juicing, there really is no place like home.

Sure, an at-home juicing machine can also be pricey and cost as much as a high-end media system (some retail for—

gasp—over $10,000). But buying a juicer is like purchasing a home—you're investing for the long-term. Grabbing your juice on the hoof can run anywhere between $2 in a super-market to $8 from a juice bar. Suddenly, going on a bender and laying out a couple of Benjamins for your own machine makes sense.

The other problem with bottled brands is that they don't always live up to their healthy hype. Juice needs to be as fresh as a just-opened bag of potato chips if you want to harvest all those five-syllable benefits like phytonutrients and antioxidants. In juice-years, anything over a day old already qualifies your drink for an AARP [formerly known as American Association of Retired Persons] card. Even if your store-bought juice was made and delivered before the sun rose, it would still be older than it appears to be because it's been pasteurized so it can age with grace. In addition, it most likely has additives to keep it looking young and vibrant, and, possibly, sugar to give it a sweeter disposition. Roll up your sleeves and do the juicing yourself and you decide exactly what goes in to make an on-the-spot health drink.

This is where cold pressing really goes to the top of the class. Rather than grinding and pulverizing the veggies and fruit, which can oxidize and degrade the nutrients, this kind of no-blade juicing process slow presses and squeezes the liquid out of the produce. This means less contact with oxygen or heat, less pulp and more liquid. The result is an easily digestible, minimally processed, thicker drink filled with healthy ingredients. . . .

If, like My Little Pony's Ranty, you're thinking green isn't your color, know that those cold press drinks are as varied, fresh, colorful and flavorful as a Mardi Gras parade. Sure, there are supergreen juices for dense doses of nutrients, but there are also fruity juices for quick, sweet jolts, nutty milk juices for a powerful protein punch, rooty vegetables with an earthy, Birkenstock undertone, blended juices DIY-designed for whatever ails you, juices that contain hemp, chlorophyll, sprouts, spirulina and/or chia seeds to supersize your antioxidant consumption, juices that offset radio-poisoning (at least, if you're Iron Man Tony Stark; for the rest of us mere mortals, the only counteraction benefit we might reap is that the motor of some juicers will drown out bad seventies rock stations), juices that taste like salad, juices that taste like candy, juices that taste like they were conceived by the Swamp Thing and juices that somehow taste like all three and are still delish.

You want to make your juice taste good—but with green veggies. If you throw in too many apples, grapes or bananas, it's like drinking a cup of sugar.

Moderation Matters

Still, it's not quite as simple as "knock back a juice, get healthy." While juicing can offer a low-fat, nutrient-rich shot of energy, like all things dietary, the benefits are reaped when it's done in moderation as opposed to as a long-term substitute for real food. Unlike smoothies or blending, juicing squeezes our fiber. However, the Harvard School of Public Health recommends that in order to keep our poop pipes running smoothly, our tummies full, our waistlines trim, our sugar levels steady and our risk of heart disease, colon cancer, high cholesterol and diabetes low, we need to put away 14 grams of fiber for every 1,000 calories of food we eat each day (for the mathematically challenged, that adds up to 28 grams for most women and 38 grams for most men). So you either need to supplement your juices with some fiber-loaded foods or work some of the pulp back into your menu. . . .

Another potential dietary hazard to keep an eye out for—and one more reason to home-juice—is making sure that your juice cup does not runneth over with sugar. Juice doesn't have to be liquid candy. You can spike it with spices or lemon juice or sweeten it with a touch of sugar, but if you don't keep the drink mainly green, you'll just be drinking some Hawaiian Punch tarted up with veggies. Just memorize this ratio: 4:1. Or, if your mind leans numerically this way, 80:20 percent. This means that for every serving of fruit, you should try to take the sweet edge off with a minimum of four servings of leafy or cruciferous vegetables. (Vegetables like beets and carrots fall into a sweet, starchy black hole and should therefore not always have the start position in your juice.) You can figure out the measurements (do your calculations before you juice) with the "What Counts?" table, but don't worry about getting it exactly right. This is a rule of thumb rather than an exact formula. After all, an orange is going to produce a lot more juice than a bunch of Romaine lettuce.

Yes, you want to make your juice taste good—but with green veggies. If you throw in too many apples, grapes or bananas, it's like drinking a cup of sugar. Even 100 percent fruit juice with no natural sweeteners added can have as much sugar and as many calories as soda. Yup, you read right. In a study published in the *Lancet Diabetes & Endocrinology*, researchers determined that one cup of apple juice contains 110 calories and a jaw-dropping 26 grams of sugar, which is almost the same as what you'd find in the same-size serving of cola.

By throwing in the odd apple or orange as a sweetener, you create a glass of healthy goodness any nutritionist would want to drink.

Fruit is naturally jam-packed with fructose, which is essentially the molecule that makes sugar sweet. On a good day, the body gets the right amount of fructose (about 15 grams, unless you have hyperuricemia or high uric acid levels). It converts this fructose to glycogen (liver starch) as a storehouse for ready energy. This can then be fished out of your liver if your body needs glucose in the future—for instance, if you've depleted your ready stock from a heavy-duty workout or you're starving (meaning you've skipped more than a few meals—getting hungry in the slump between lunch and dinner doesn't count). So that's how it should work.

But more commonly, we feed our bodies too much fructose—and it's hard not to since it's in practically everything from agave syrup to tortilla chips to chocolate bars to raw pistachio nuts. A National Institutes of Health (NIH) study determined that the average American diet weighs in at 37+ grams of fructose daily. The problem is, too much fructose and our digestive system—specifically the liver—becomes overwhelmed and unable to process it fast enough for the body to use a sugar.

Sure, the sugar from that soda is processed and the sugar from produce is Mama Nature's best. But it actually makes no difference if the fructose is from too much fruit or too much junk food—all fructose works the same in the body. Like that out-of-control conveyor belt from the classic *I Love Lucy* candy factory episode, the liver goes haywire and starts making fats from the fructose and sending them into the bloodstream as triglycerides (a type of fat or lipid in your blood and an important measure of heart health). This can have a three-pronged effect: 1) substantially increased risk of heart disease, high cholesterol, liver disease, some cancers and gout; 2) since the fructose does an end run around the body's appetite signal system, the mind doesn't register that it's full, which leads to overeating and weight gain; and 3) screaming panic headlines tarring fruit juice as a major cause for type 2 diabetes risk (British Medical Association) and worse for you than a Krispy Kreme donut (Credit Suisse Research Institute).

However, there's no danger in juicing and there are a load of benefits as long as you stick to the 4:1 ratio. Giving the vegetables the starring role and the fruit a bit part in your juice means you'll also soften some of the stronger flavors of those mega-healthy greens. By throwing in the odd apple or orange as a sweetener, you create a glass of healthy goodness any nutritionist would want to drink. In this mix, homemade juice truly becomes the ultimate convenience food: You don't even have to chew, or, in many cases, cook. You just have it your way.

11

Juicing Can Be Harmful to Health

Diane Wedner

Diane Wedner is a health writer for Lifescript, a website focusing on women's health, and former reporter for the Los Angeles Times.

Fresh vegetable and fruit juices may be the new "latte," but juicing too much can be unhealthy and even dangerous. The high vitamin K content in spinach-kale smoothies can be life-threatening to those taking blood-thinning medications, and high servings of fruit each day can lead to the development of diabetes. Also, juices with high potassium ingredients can damage the kidneys, and those with greens such as kale, spinach, and collards may threaten the thyroid gland. Moreover, juices are ineffective in cleanses, can be high in calories, and deprive the diet of fiber, which helps the colon and lowers cholesterol and blood sugar levels.

You just stumbled out of yoga class. You're hot, sweaty and need a pick-me-up. Go for a nonfat latte? No, you grab a kale juice instead.

Juice is now the beverage of choice for people on the go. Harried moms drink it. So do yoga fans. Celebrities Gwyneth Paltrow, Jared Leto and Salma Hayek do too.

They're juicing—chugging raw fruit-and-vegetable drinks to "cleanse" their bodies, get a speedy meal, consume more produce or lose weight.

Juice is the new latte. About 92 million gallons of super-premium juices were consumed in 2013, up from 71 million gallons in 2007, according to Beverage Marketing Corp., an industry research firm.

No wonder! Juice is an easy way to get fresh vegetables and fruit. It makes for a fast breakfast or lunch, and it's healthful.

Or is it? Could something this good be bad for you?

Yes, especially if you have a chronic condition or are taking certain drugs, says Adrienne Youdim, M.D., assistant professor of medicine and medical director of the Center for Weight Loss at Cedars-Sinai Medical Center in Los Angeles.

If you take anticoagulants, you should only eat a half-cup of leafy greens a day, according to the National Institutes of Health Clinical Center.

Even if you're a healthy person, too much juice can be dangerous, warns nutrition expert Carol Koprowski, Ph.D., R.D., assistant professor of clinical preventive medicine at Keck School of Medicine of USC [University of Southern California] in Los Angeles. So before grabbing a carrot juice instead of lunch or spending hundreds on a cleanse, read on for the 8 ways juicing can hurt you. . . .

1. You Could Risk Dangerous Drug Interactions

The high vitamin K content in a spinach-kale smoothie, for example, can be life-threatening if you take blood-thinning medications, like warfarin. Such anticoagulants often are prescribed after a stroke, deep vein thrombosis or other circulatory conditions.

Kale, spinach, turnip greens, collards, Swiss chard, parsley and mustard greens—green juicers' favorites—contain up to 550 micrograms of vitamin K per cup, which can lower the drugs' anti-clotting activity.

If you take anticoagulants, you should only eat a half-cup of leafy greens a day, according to the National Institutes of Health Clinical Center. Eat the same amount every day too, because big changes in vitamin K intake could lead to a blood clot, and a stroke or death. If you're one of the 70 million people taking cholesterol-lowering statins, stay away from grapefruit juice. The citrus fruit blocks an intestinal enzyme that controls absorption of drugs such as simvastatin or ator-vastatin.

You'll also face a higher risk of muscle and joint pain, muscle breakdown, liver damage and kidney failure if you drink grapefruit juice (or eat the fruit) while taking statins, according to the Cleveland Clinic.

Grapefruit also can interfere with drugs for high blood pressure, anxiety, allergies and other ailments, according to the Food and Drug Administration. So ask your doctor if your prescriptions may interact with the fruit.

2. You Could Develop Diabetes

About 79 million Americans have prediabetes, according to the American Diabetes Association.

That means they have blood sugar readings that are higher than healthy but not yet high enough for a diabetes diagnosis. Juicing could tip those at risk over the edge, according to a 2010 Harvard University study of 187,000 nurses.

Drinking one or more daily servings of apple, orange, grapefruit and other juices increases the risk of developing type 2 diabetes by 21%, the study found.

If you have the metabolic disorder, juicing could lead to blood sugar spikes because you're getting all the sugar of fruit without the fiber, Koprowski explains. The fiber in whole fruit and vegetables slows the absorption of sugar into the bloodstream. If you've been told you have prediabetes, eat the whole fruit instead. But limit daily intake to one small piece of fruit or one cup of fresh berries or melon, Koprowski advises.

3. You Could Damage Your Kidneys

Beware of fruit and vegetable juices with high amounts of potassium, such as bananas and kale, if you have kidney problems.

Four-and-a-half cups of chopped kale—the amount in 8 ounces of juice for a "cleanse"—can be lethal if your kidneys are weak because of high blood pressure, severe infection, an enlarged prostate, certain drugs or pregnancy complications.

Even most lower-potassium foods are off-limits to people with kidney problems because the amounts add up quickly.

Adults need 4,700 mg of potassium daily to keep the heart and muscles working. In healthy people, the kidneys generally excrete the excess. But that doesn't happen in people with compromised kidneys: Potassium builds in their blood, raising the risk of a heart attack and stroke, according to the National Kidney Foundation. They should limit their intake of potassium to 1,500–2,000 mg per day.

> *Even most lower-potassium foods are off-limits to people with kidney problems because the amounts add up quickly.*

If you have experienced weakness, numbness or tingling—signs of potassium overload—call your doctor immediately, advises Judy D. Simon, M.S., R.D., a clinical dietitian and nutritionist at the University of Washington Medical Center's Roosevelt Clinic in Seattle.

4. You Could Threaten Your Thyroid Gland

Kale, bok choy, cauliflower, collards and spinach are rich in glucosinolates, which form goitrin, a compound associated with hypothyroidism or insufficient thyroid hormone.

High amounts of these veggies have caused hypothyroidism in animals, according to Oregon State University's Linus Pauling Institute. One 88-year-old woman lapsed into a coma after eating 3 pounds (or 2 cups of juice) per day of raw bok choy for several months, according to the institute. But researchers aren't sure if her condition was caused by the bok choy or another problem, such as an autoimmune disease.

The National Cancer Institute recommends eating a variety of vegetables daily—not just leafy green ones. The CDC's [Centers for Disease Control and Prevention] fruit-and-veggie calculator helps you determine how much you need. But there are no separate intake recommendations for people with hypothyroidism, so talk to your doctor before juicing.

5. You Might Get Food Poisoning

One reason fresh juice is healthful is that it's unpasteurized, so the taste and nutrients are preserved.

But when juices aren't heated to 154°F for 30 minutes to kill germs, they're more vulnerable to lethal bacteria, such as salmonella, *Listeria monocytogenes* and *Toxoplasma gondii*, according to the Centers for Disease Control and Prevention (CDC).

Even if it's bacteria-free during manufacturing, fresh juice sold in stores may be contaminated after it leaves the plant— for example, in shipping, storage or in your home.

Forget about [juice cleanses]. The practice is a waste of time and money, because your body doesn't need "cleansing."

If you leave a container of juice on a table overnight, toss it. Otherwise you risk food poisoning and major intestinal problems, the U.S. Department of Agriculture warns.

Most store-bought, bottled fresh juices last up to 3 days if refrigerated and unopened, Koprowski says. Drink them within a day once you've opened the seal.

Flash-pasteurizing—heating juice at 160° for 15–30 seconds—offers a longer shelf life, about 3 weeks in the fridge, while preserving some nutrients. Companies such as Naked Juice and Odwalla treat their juices this way. Products that aren't pasteurized must say so on the package.

6. Juice Cleanses Don't Work

We clean out our houses and cars. So why not our bodies? That's the reasoning behind juice cleanses, which are intended to rid your body of toxins. Forget about it. The practice is a waste of time and money, because your body doesn't need "cleansing," says Dr. Youdim of Cedars-Sinai.

"Our bodies have their own elaborate, elegant detoxification system, called the liver, intestines and kidneys," she explains.

"It's foolish to think the body can't detox on its own," she adds.

7. Juices Can Be Calorie Bombs

If you're downing up to 96 ounces of juice a day to lose weight—which many fasts recommend—stop, USC's Koprowski warns. Juicing for days to lose weight "can be potentially harmful," she says. That's because you're losing out on important nutrients.

And don't expect to get slimmer, says Dr. Youdim. In fact, you might gain weight, because you're consuming more calories than you realize—mostly from naturally occurring sugar in the fruits and vegetables.

Some juices and smoothies are more caloric than a meal. For example, a large Jamba Juice Razzmatazz Smoothie, made with mixed berry juice, orange sherbet, strawberries and bananas, rings up at 580 calories.

Consume too many, and "you can end up with a few thousand calories of juice a day!" Simon warns.

And still be unsatisfied.

"It can take 10–15 oranges or several pounds of carrots to make a meal of juice," Koprowski says. "Or you could munch on a couple of carrots and feel full."

8. You're Passing on Protein

Eight ounces of kale juice is packed with vitamins A (3,500% of your daily recommended amount), K (4,300%) and C (1,200%), plus iron, calcium and antioxidants. But you'll get only about 2 to 8 grams of protein.

That's not enough if you're drinking juice as a meal replacement. A 130-pound woman needs 65 grams of protein daily to repair cells and create new ones.

Juicing gives you the nutrients of fresh produce—but removes the pulp and fiber necessary to keep your colon in good working order, reduce heart disease risk, and lower cholesterol and blood sugar levels.

Protein also preserves and builds lean body mass, which helps keep you healthy and even burns calories, Dr. Youdim explains.

"Fruits and vegetables [alone], however, are not a great source," Koprowski says.

9. You're Forsaking Fiber

Juicing gives you the nutrients of fresh produce—but removes the pulp and fiber necessary to keep your colon in good working order, reduce heart disease risk, and lower cholesterol and blood sugar levels.

"When you drink orange juice, you get vitamin C, but it's not the same as eating an orange," Simon says.

The whole fruit has the vitamin plus fiber, with far fewer calories than a glass of juice. It'll also keep you full longer.

10. You'll Pay Premium Prices

A daily juice habit is expensive—about $3,500 yearly if you buy one a day from a premium juice bar. Lifescript checked around at local stores and found that:

- Evolution Fresh costs $2.99 to $6.99 for a 15-ounce bottle at Starbucks.

- You'll pay $5.99 to $9.99 for the fresh juice bar at Whole Foods.

- Premium juice bars in Los Angeles charge $10 to $15 for 8-ounce refreshers.

Cleanses are even costlier. Actress Salma Hayek's Cooler Cleanse, sold online, runs $58 per day—or $174 for 3 days of fruits, vegetables, coconut water and almond milk.

The bottom line: Juices are better than a burger and fries, and can be a good addition to your diet—if you're healthy and consume them in moderation.

"But if you want to live a healthy life and prevent chronic diseases without spending a fortune, eat whole vegetables and grains, not 'detox' protocols," Dr. Youdim advises.

Organizations to Contact

The editors have compiled the following list of organizations concerned with the issues debated in this book. The descriptions are derived from materials provided by the organizations. All have publications or information available for interested readers. The list was compiled on the date of publication of the present volume; the information provided here may change. Be aware that many organizations take several weeks or longer to respond to inquiries, so allow as much time as possible.

American Nutrition Association (ANA)

PO Box 262, Western Springs, IL   60558

website: http://americannutritionassociation.org

A nonprofit, the American Nutrition Association (ANA) began in 1972 as the Nutrition for Optimal Health Association (NOHA). Its mission is to promote optimal health through nutrition and wellness education. With science-based nutrition, ANA educates both laypeople and professionals about the health benefits of nutrition and wellness. It publishes a newsletter, *Nutrition Digest*, and offers information on health issues and nutrition at its website.

European Food Information Council (EUFIC)

Tassel House, Paul-Emile JANSON 6, Brussels   1000
   Belgium

website: www.eufic.org

Founded in 1995, the European Food Information Council (EUFIC) is a nonprofit organization that aims to help better inform consumers in choosing well-balanced, safe, and healthy eating habits and lifestyle. It offers publications on food issues and a newsletter, *Food Today*, online.

Food and Agriculture Organization of the United Nations (FAO)

Viale delle Terme di Caracalla, Rome   00153
  Italy
+39 06 57051
e-mail: fao-hq@fao.org
website: www.fao.org

The main goals of the Food and Agriculture Organization of the United Nations (FAO) are the eradication of hunger, food insecurity, and malnutrition; the elimination of poverty and the driving forward of economic and social progress for all; and the sustainable management and utilization of natural resources, including land, water, air, climate, and genetic resources for the benefit of present and future generations. It organized 2013's "International Year of Quinoa" and offers information on various superfoods at its website.

Food Matters

PO Box 1302, Mooloolaba   QLD 4557
  Australia
website: http://foodmatters.tv

James Colquhoun and Laurentine ten Bosch are directors of Food Matters, a website based on the 2008 documentary created by the couple to educate people about the benefits of natural health. Their website offers information on superfoods as well as articles, videos, and guides on nutrition and natural health.

International Blueberry Organization (IBO)

website: www.internationalblueberry.org

The International Blueberry Organization (IBO) is a global entity bringing together leaders from around the blueberry world in all segments of the industry. The organization works to increase understanding and purvey information, to address mutual challenges and coordinate potential solutions, and to explore opportunities. Its website offers information on the health benefits of blueberries.

National Kale Day
2109 Broadway, Suite 5-20, New York, NY   10023
(201) 345-6789
website: http://nationalkaleday.org

National Kale Day advocates kale as a vegetable with incredible health benefits and culinary versatility. The first inaugural National Kale Day was held in October 2013. Its website provides nutritional information on kale as well as recipes and resources.

US Department of Agriculture (USDA)
1400 Independence Ave. SW, Washington, DC   20250
(202) 720-2791
website: www.usda.gov

The US Department of Agriculture (USDA) aims to expand economic opportunity through innovation, helping rural America to thrive; to promote agriculture production sustainability that better nourishes Americans while also helping feed others throughout the world; and to preserve and conserve the nation's natural resources through restored forests, improved watersheds, and healthy private working lands. The USDA website covers topics such as food, nutrition, and organic agriculture.

Whole Grains Council
266 Beacon St., Boston, MA   02116
(617) 421-5500 • fax: (617) 421-5511
website: http://wholegrainscouncil.org

The Whole Grains Council is a nonprofit consumer advocacy group working to increase consumption of whole grains for better health. The council's many initiatives include encouraging manufacturers to create delicious whole grain products, helping consumers to find whole grain foods and understand their health benefits, and helping the media to write accurate, compelling stories about whole grains. On its website, it offers a "Whole Grains 101" section with information on superfoods.

World Health Organization (WHO)

Ave. Appia 20, Geneva 27   1211
  Switzerland
+41 22 791 21 11 • fax: +41 22 791 31 11
e-mail: info@who.int
website: www.who.int

The World Health Organization (WHO) is the directing and coordinating authority for health within the United Nations (UN) system. It is responsible for providing leadership on global health matters, shaping the health research agenda, setting norms and standards, articulating evidence-based policy options, providing technical support to countries, and monitoring and assessing health trends. Online, WHO provides information on nutrition, diet, and nutritional disorders.

Bibliography

Books

Bob Arnot

The Aztec Diet: Chia Power: The Superfood That Gets You Skinny and Keeps You Healthy. New York: William Morrow, 2013.

Lauri Boone

Powerful Plant-Based Superfoods: The Best Way to Eat for Maximum Health, Energy, and Weight Loss. Minneapolis, MN: Fair Winds Press, 2013.

Elliot Lang

Eating Insects. Eating Insects as Food. Dublin, Ireland: IMB Publishing, 2013.

Michael Murray

The Complete Book of Juicing: Your Delicious Guide to Youthful Vitality. New York: Clarkson Potter, 2013.

Michael T. Murray, Joseph Pizzorno, and Lara Pizzorno

The Encyclopedia of Healing Foods. New York: Atria Books, 2005.

Stephanie Pedersen

Kale: The Complete Guide to the World's Most Powerful Superfood. New York: Sterling, 2013.

Steven G. Pratt

SuperFoods RX: Fourteen Foods That Will Change Your Life. New York: Harper, 2006.

Drew Ramsey and Jennifer Iserloh

Fifty Shades of Kale: 50 Fresh and Satisfying Recipes That Are Bound to Please. New York: HarperWave, 2013.

Tonia Reinhard   *Superfoods: The Healthiest Foods on the Planet*. Richmond Hill, Ontario, Canada: Firefly Books Limited, 2014.

Alexander G. Schauss   *Acai: An Extraordinary Antioxidant-Rich Palm Fruit from the Amazon*. Tacoma, WA: BioSocial Publications, 2006.

Periodicals and Internet Sources

Emma Beckett and Zoe Yates   "Superfoods: Not So Super After All?," The Conversation, June 16, 2013. http://theconversation.com.

Sarah Berry   "Dissecting Pete Evans' Diet," *Sydney Morning Herald*, November 13, 2012.

Melissa Breyer   "Superfoods: 11 Berries to Improve Your Health," Mother Nature Network, April 26, 2013. www.mnn.com.

Michael Casey   "Bugs in Your Protein Bar: Are Edible Insects the Next Food Craze?," *Fortune*, July 18, 2014.

Stephanie Castillo   "Don't Get Duped By These So-Called Superfoods; What's Really Worth Buying in the Grocery Store," *Medical Daily*, August 30, 2014.

Tom Chivers   "The Myth of the 'Superfood,'" *Telegraph*, October 13, 2014.

Tim Ferriss   "10 Uncommon 'Superfoods' from the World of Ultra-Endurance," *Huffington Post*, May 31, 2013. www.huffingtonpost.com.

Melanie Haiken

"The Next Miracle Superfood: Insects, Scientists Say," *Forbes*, July 11, 2014.

Melissa McEwen

"Just Kale Me: How Your Kale Habit Is Slowly Destroying Your Health and the World," Hunt Gather Love, August 31, 2013. http://huntgatherlove.com,

Bess O'Connor

"Move Over Acai Berries: The Next Wave of Superfoods Is Here," MindBodyGreen, December 4, 2014. www.mindbodygreen.com.

Jen Schwartz

"Striving for the Perfect Diet Is Making Us Sick," *Popular Science*, February 5, 2015.

Larry Schwartz

"8 Superfoods That Aren't All That Super," *AlterNet*, September 26, 2014. www.alternet.org.

Elaine Sciolino

"Trendy Green Mystifies France. It's a Job for the Kale Crusader!," *New York Times*, September 21, 2013.

Index

A

AARP (American Association of Retired Persons), 79
Açai, 43
Acid-neutralizing minerals, 61
Adair Kitchen, 46
Adib, Racha, 7, 8
African Mango, 14–15
Alcohol consumption, 25, 30
Alzheimer's disease, 77
Amaranth, 7
Amasai, 13
American Diabetes Association, 86
American Journal of Clinical Nutrition, 17
American Journal of Epidemiology, 76
American Journal of Medicine, 77
Amylase enzyme, 15
Andean farmers, 64–65
Andean Information Network, 66
Andean Naturals, 65
Antebi, Marcus, 43, 46, 47
Anthrocyanins, 51–55
Anticarcinogenic activity, 52
Anti-clotting activity, 86
Anti-inflammatory foods, 44, 45
Antimicrobial compounds, 52
Antioxidants, 42, 44, 50–53
Arizona Center for Integrative Medicine, 8
Aronia (chokeberries) berries, 52, 55
Atorvastatin, 86
Axe, Josh, 10–19

B

Backhouse, Tasneem, 40
Bale, Christian, 17
Ban Ki-moon, 67
Banks, Emma, 66, 69
Baobab fruit, 9
Barnard, Nick, 40
Barnhart, Katie Adair, 46
Beetroot, 24, 35, 52
Behind the Headlines, 25
Beverage Marketing Corp., 85
Bioflavanoids, 18
Black tea, 27
Blood glucose, 15
Blueberries, 44
Body mass index (BMI), 29
Bolling, Bill, 49–55
Breast cancer, 11–12, 14
British Medical Journal, 19
Broccoli, 22, 23, 26, 33
Buffalo berries, 35

C

Cacao, 47–48
Calcium, 61
Cancer
    anticarcinogenic activity, 52
    breast cancer, 11–12, 14
    follow-up period in research, 28
    introduction, 10
Cardiovascular risks/health, 33–34
Carotenoids, 53
Casein proteins, 61

99